Feeling Machines

FEELING MACHINES

Japanese Robotics
and the Global Entanglements
of More-Than-Human Care

SHAWN BENDER

STANFORD UNIVERSITY PRESS
Stanford, California

Stanford University Press
Stanford, California

Printed in the United States of America on acid-free, archival-quality paper

Library of Congress Cataloging-in-Publication Data
Names: Bender, Shawn Morgan, author.
Title: Feeling machines : Japanese robotics and the global entanglements of
    more-than-human care / Shawn Bender.
Description: Stanford, California : Stanford University Press, 2024. | Includes
    bibliographical references and index.
Identifiers: LCCN 2024009281 (print) | LCCN 2024009282 (ebook)
    | ISBN 9781503640191 (cloth) | ISBN 9781503641150 (paperback) |
    ISBN 9781503641167 (ebook)
Subjects: LCSH: Robotics in medicine—Social aspects. | Robots—Therapeutic
    use. | Human-robot interaction. | Robotics—Human factors. | Older people—
    Care—Technological innovations. | People with disabilities—Care—
    Technological innovations. | Robotics—Japan.
Classification: LCC R857.R63 B46 2024 (print) | LCC R857.R63 (ebook) |
    DDC 610.2856—dc23/eng/20240528
LC record available at https://lccn.loc.gov/2024009281
LC ebook record available at https://lccn.loc.gov/2024009282

Cover design: Bob Aufuldish, Aufuldish & Warinner
Cover art: US Patent & Trademark Office #8511964

CONTENTS

LIST OF ILLUSTRATIONS

PREFACE

Life in the Loop

The future is just a half-step away.

Somewhere in Japan a high school girl awakens to a voice coming from the smartphone next to her pillow. She bolts upright and turns toward the window, letting her eyes adjust to the glare of the morning sun. "A package is arriving in ten minutes," the voice says. She hurries downstairs and steps onto a wide veranda overlooking a small vegetable field. A white quadcopter drone approaches and hovers just a few feet above her head. The drone scans her face, confirms her identity, and drops a small box into her hands. "Right on time!" she thinks to herself. She steps back inside her house, admiring the new pair of sneakers in the box.

Now dressed for school, the girl walks into her kitchen and asks her refrigerator what she should have for breakfast. The machine suggests a smoothie and displays a recipe on its LED screen. She sits down to enjoy it. Moments later, a speaker in the room reminds the girl that it's time to leave for school. She tells the speaker to order her two sandwiches "at the usual place." Hurrying out the door, she yells goodbye to her grandmother in the next room. "See you later," grandmother calls after her. Grandmother turns back to the computer in front of her. A doctor on screen says that her blood pressure has been high for the past couple of days. "Oh, really?" she worries out loud.

Now outside, granddaughter runs to the grocery store with her brand-new sneakers on, book bag bouncing off her hip. Lush green mountains rise up along the horizon. Wires stretch between tall electric transmission towers in front of them. A self-driving tractor harvests rice in a patty next to the road. The girl arrives at the store to pick up her order. She breathlessly greets the cashier. Tapping her phone on a touchpad, she pays for her order and dashes back outside.

Now she waits at a bus stop. "Phew! Made it just in time," an older boy mumbles to himself as he jogs up next to her. The girl turns to him, and her expression changes in an instant—this is someone she likes. She looks down. He's wearing the same sneakers that she is! "Hi," she says with a smile. "Ah, you're riding, too?" the boy responds flatly.

A self-driving bus stops in front of them. They board together and find seats at the back. They are now visible through the rear windshield. They sit together, laughing and talking. The girl turns away from the boy. She looks out the window toward us, toward the camera. "The future looks fun, doesn't it?" *(mirai ga tanoshimi desho?)*, she says. The scene cuts to an idyllic rural landscape framed in a stationary shot. The name of this future scrolls across a cloudless sky.

Society 5.0. Coming soon . . .

————————

What may seem like an ad for a futuristic teen romance is actually a promotional video that appeared in 2017 on a website run by the Government of Japan. The government produced the video in order to dramatize the central elements of "Society 5.0," its vision of a future in which ubiquitous "smart" machines, artificial intelligence systems, Big Data analytics, and robotics combine to usher forth a new epoch in Japan—the era of the "super smart society" *(chō sumāto shakai)*. Society 5.0, which the government first detailed in the country's Fifth Science and Technology Basic Plan in 2015, is part of a package of economic reforms, known colloquially as "Abenomics," initiated by then prime minister Abe Shinzō.[1] Amid a set of policies directed at the economy, the emphasis on *society* in this plan should not be minimized. The "super smart society" of Society 5.0 is not intended only to foster economic growth. The super smart society aims to solve social problems as well (see figure P.1).

Chief among these problems, one that underlies nearly every aspect of

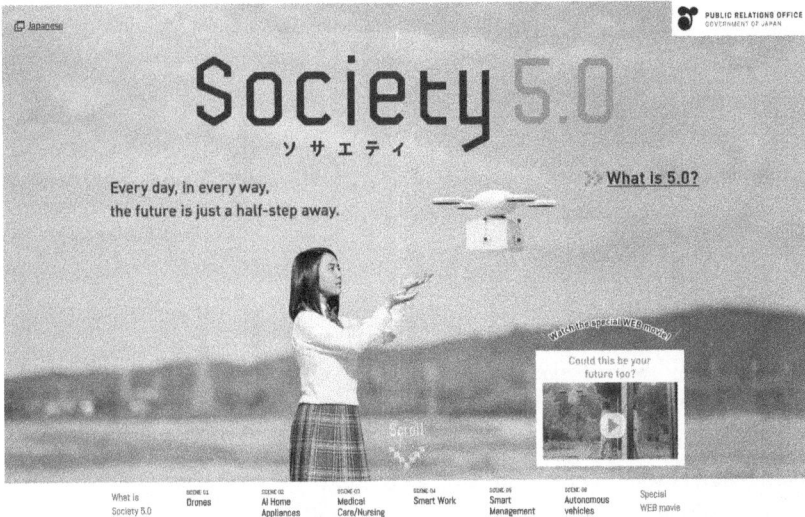

FIGURE P.1 The Future Vision of Society 5.0. A screenshot of the Japanese government's website for Society 5.0, its vision of a future sustained by ubiquitous smart technologies. Source: Official Website of the Prime Minister of Japan and His Cabinet (https://www.gov-online.go.jp/cam/s5/index.html).

Society 5.0 solutionism, is population aging. Japan currently has the largest proportion of seniors in the world and among the lowest levels of fertility. The impact of a rising number of seniors on the health and welfare services of the state, especially in light of projected labor shortages, has long been a concern of political and industrial elites in Japan (Robertson 2018; Wright 2023). The technologies fueling Society 5.0 are intended in large part to soften the impact of the "low birthrate, aging society" *(shōshi kōreika shakai)* on a future Japan.

Consider the setting of the video. This is not a sleek megalopolis of cyberpunk imagination. This is the Japanese countryside, where low birthrates and youth out-migration have led to population aging at rates far exceeding municipalities. Where there are fewer people, the intelligent machines of Society 5.0 will fill the void. No workers available to bring your new shoes? An autonomous drone will do it for you. No mother around to make you breakfast? Your smart fridge will find you a recipe. No farmers around to plant and harvest foods like rice? A robotic tractor will do it for you. No drivers ready to take the kids to school? An autonomous bus will drive them for you. No one around to take care of grandma? Machines will alert doctors when something is amiss. Machines won't threaten our survival; they will enable it. They will care for us!

In proposing technological solutions to pressing societal problems in Japan, Society 5.0 is hardly novel. A decade earlier, the first Abe government (2006–7) outlined *Innovation 25*, a picture of what Japan would look like in 2025 should it aggressively develop robots for everyday use. *Innovation 25* assured citizens that the fundamental basis of everyday life would be conserved even in the face of considerable technological change and intensifying demographic pressure. As the anthropologist Jennifer Robertson writes, "[In *Innovation 25*] the declining birth rate, labor shortage, and rapidly aging population are . . . treated in large part as problems that can be 'fixed' by technological solutions" (Robertson 2018, 19).

Society 5.0, too, depicts technology as a fix for anticipated demographic change. But continuity of purpose does not necessarily entail similarity in substance. In *Innovation 25*, it is humanoid robots—robots that look and act human—that cook, clean, and take care of children and the elderly. In Society 5.0, by contrast, humanoid robots are conspicuously absent. Everyday objects—phones, fridges, speakers, tractors, buses—have instead been roboticized. These ambient technologies recede into the background. They "think" and interact with the analog (and digital) world just as a humanoid robot might, yet they maintain a superficial appearance that is decidedly nonhuman(oid). In fact, many of them are already here: Amazon proposed delivery drones years ago; smartphones already notify users of impending deliveries; smart speakers can already place orders for their owners; and self-driving tractors, cars, and buses are in development worldwide. The future portrayed in Society 5.0 is not just imaginable, it is virtually here. This is a future realized through the gradual *iteration* of everyday technologies, updates from version 1.0 to 2.0 all the way to 5.0. Indeed, the government website tells us: *Every day, in every way, the future is just a half-step away.*

Yet, as much as the smart machines of Society 5.0 might appear ready to serve *us*, they also depend on us. They function by tracking our actions and sensing shifts in our moods and desires. An illustration on the Cabinet Office website for Society 5.0 depicts life in this near future (figure P.2). At its center, three generations of a family stand together inside a circle glowing blue. Four text bubbles distributed along the circle display the names of technologies that are vital to the super smart future: "IoT [Internet of Things],"

Realizing Society 5.0

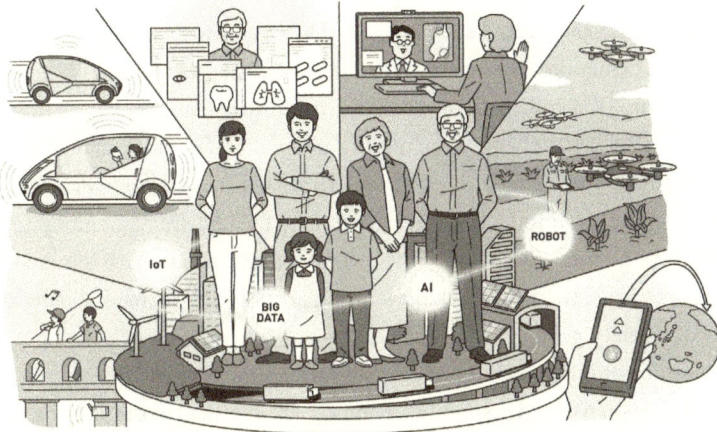

FIGURE P.2 Loops of Life. Promotional image from a Japanese government website for Society 5.0 shows Family, Society, Nature, and Industry supported by the feedback loops that animate networked technologies. Source: Official Website of the Prime Minister of Japan and His Cabinet (https://www.japan.go.jp/abenomics/_userdata/abenomics/pdf/society_5.0.pdf).

"Big Data," "AI," "Robot." Below the family is a round plot of green grass dotted with homes, office buildings, solar panels, and wind turbines. Along the perimeter, electric trucks drive along a highway that curves around the grassy area, forming yet another circle.

The meaning of the imagery seems clear enough: the cyclical rhythms of digitally enabled material infrastructures are the (literal) ground on which the family of the future will stand. Family—the fundamental unit of Japanese society, under threat of fragmentation by the forces of demographic change—will be sustained, just as nature will be protected and culture preserved. Still, humans remain at the center. The machines rely on us much as we might rely on them. Without human behavior to track, to analyze, to optimize, the feedback loops of Society 5.0 would not spin at all.

Over a decade ago, when I began studying the everyday use of Japanese "care robots" *(kaigo robotto)*, I did not expect that my research would come to focus on the kinds of feedback loops that would animate the imagination of Society 5.0 years later. Care robots emerged in Japan through efforts to engineer technologies for the "aging society," but they have since been integrated into the care of dementia and disability in locations around the world. They are a special kind of robot. Unlike industrial machines, care robots are intended for direct, often tactile, engagement with people. In fact, they rarely work independently of such interactions. They are what I call *feeling machines*; that is, robots engineered to feel and designed to be felt. Feeling machines depend on and respond to feedback generated in direct interaction with human users. In these respects, their functionality anticipates the roboticized objects at the center of Society 5.0.

Relations of feedback are, of course, fundamental to the operation of any robot. Robots sense and respond to events in the physical world only by means of continuous loops of feedback flowing from sensors to processing units, from processing units out to mechanical actuators, and then back again. But, as I observed care robots at work in multiple sites, I heard feedback described additionally as the main mechanism by which feeling machines facilitate care delivery. Among older adults with dementia, for example, care workers told me how engaging with feeling machines generates positive feelings and enhances quality of life beyond what interactions with human care workers can accomplish alone. Among patients with walking disabilities, therapists explained how a robotic exoskeleton could "heal through feedback" by interfacing directly with the body and amplifying nerve signals flowing between brain and limb. Crucially, such relations of feedback were not confined to therapeutic encounters. Robotics researchers and robot makers relied on everyday practices of care to provide vital feedback on the operational successes and failures of their machines. Local and national governments similarly sponsored opportunities to interact with care robots as a means of revealing potential markets for care and other technologies in the future. Feeling machines, I found, generate(s) overlapping relations of feedback that facilitate practices of care in the present and direct processes of innovation into the future.

In this book, I follow the loops of feedback set in motion by the flow of Japanese feeling machines around the world to better understand the relationship of technology to care and the relationship of care to technology.

In so doing, I analyze the relations that care robots afford through a lens drawn from the world of technology development itself. I use the term *iterative engagements* to refer to generative encounters with feeling machines. This framing derives from a now-dominant "iterative" approach to software development that relies on real-time user feedback, defers finality, foregoes functional perfection, and integrates operational failure within processes of creation. Iterative development is anti-teleological; it aims less at utopic perfection than at endless, incremental increases in functionality (Bialski 2020). In an era of ubiquitous internet and mobile technology, iterative approaches have begun to guide the development of hardware that depends on software to function.

Approaching the study of care robotics as iterative engagement attends to the affectively charged futurity enacted by an economy of feeling machines. It centers the processual dimensions of the digital economy—how we are transformed in everyday interaction with digital devices that are transformed in their interactions with us. It aligns the small field of care robotics with government techno-solutionism and growing consumer demand for more intelligent, more responsive, and more useful digital machines. Studying care robotics as iterative engagement, then, does not just reveal new, more-than-human relations of care for older adults and persons with disabilities. It draws attention to the shifting ontologies of digital technology and to their impact on us as techno-social beings. It thus extends recent anthropological efforts to "[think] *with*, not just *about*, technology" (Fisch 2019, 6, emphasis in original) by privileging temporality and process in the analysis of robot technology.[2]

Whether Society 5.0 is actually realized is less significant, I propose, than the way in which it has been imagined, for visions of the future are arguably always about the present. Society 5.0 embraces iteration as both a metaphor for and a mechanism of the future. The vision represents contemporary "life in the loop" to Japanese as a future to which they should aspire and by which they will be reassured. Still, it is people who remain at the center of a cascade of digital feedback loops. Their future unfolds together with feeling machines encountered here or there, or maybe someday, in the process of becoming otherwise.

Care Robotics 1.0

Someday.

Minoru Murata[1] sat on the edge of the bed in his living room, nibbling on a rice cracker he had just picked from the table of food in front of us. He leaned forward and raised an eyebrow.

"Sounds great. When can I get one?"

I couldn't answer. I had no idea.

We were sitting together on a frigid January day not long after the New Year's festivities of 2011 and only a few months into my sabbatical research on robotics technologies for eldercare in Japan. During this time, I lived on the second floor of the Murata home in western Tokyo in a room that Minoru and his wife, Keiko, both in their seventies, had rented to overseas researchers for years. We chatted occasionally as I came and went but we had precious few opportunities to talk. The slower pace of life around the new year, customarily a time for family gatherings, finally gave us a chance to get acquainted.

A few years before we met, Minoru suffered a cerebral aneurysm that left him with only partial use of the right side of his body. Since he could no longer manage the steep stairs that led to the second floor of the house, the couple relocated to the living space on the first floor, which they had originally rented to tenants. Now confined to a bed that had been moved into

1

the living room, Minoru relied on his wife to help him with everyday tasks. His lack of mobility was a source of some frustration. Before the aneurysm, the Muratas had loved traveling abroad. They also enjoyed socializing with friends and colleagues, or with the foreign scholars they hosted. This was the worst thing, he would often say. He sorely missed the taste of beer and sake.

Encouraged by him nonetheless, I sheepishly took a sip of beer and sampled the many dishes Keiko had prepared for all of us. I looked up and met his gaze.

"It's not ready yet. Unfortunately, you'll have to wait."

We were talking about my trip to a robotics manufacturer in neighboring Ibaraki Prefecture. I had recently visited the showroom of a company that makes the robot HAL, a wearable exoskeleton meant to help those with partial paralysis of the limbs regain some mobility. By means of strategically placed sensors that adhere to the surface of the wearer's skin, the exoskeleton detects faint electrical traces of nerve signals as they travel to the extremities from the brain. These signals are processed in real time by a computer housed in a module on the waistband of the exoskeleton. The computer then triggers motorized joints on the hips and knees that, in combination with an additional system of sensors, support the movement intended by the person wearing it.

On my visit, a young associate in the showroom placed sensors on my right bicep and forearm. As I moved my arm up and down, part of the exoskeleton moved along with me. "Now watch this," he said, smiling in anticipation of my response. I lifted my arm up again but this time he held my forearm and told me to keep pushing. To my surprise, the robotic arm continued upward as it had before. Holding my arm was an action meant to simulate a physical impairment.

It was a demonstration meant to amaze and amaze me it did. But it was only a demonstration. Despite the glitzy showroom in which it was presented, the HAL exoskeleton was not salable to consumers for personal use. It was available only for lease and at a cost out of the reach of most individual consumers. Additionally, at the time, its safety had yet to be scientifically verified. Rather than individual elderly, its target markets were institutions like hospitals and nursing homes. Only in such places could such a new device be closely monitored, studied, adjusted, and later improved.

Like so many robots I encountered that year, it was not yet ready.

Mr. Murata looked at me, agitated. "Well, tell them to hurry up and make something I can use!"

I nodded. I understood his frustration.

———

Elsewhere.

"If you really want to see how people use my robot, you should go to Denmark."

In summer 2009, Dr. Takanori Shibata and I met in the lobby restaurant of an Osaka hotel. Shibata is a kinetic presence. He has a quick mind, speaks rapidly, and always seems in a hurry for another appointment. In fact, he usually does have another appointment. He is the inventor of Paro, a furry white robot that looks like a baby harp seal and responds to speech and touch. At the time that I met him, Shibata had been developing iterations of Paro for over a decade. Fluent in English, he often travels internationally to present research on the therapeutic benefits of his robot and to promote its adoption. I felt fortunate to have the opportunity to meet him in person.

His robot Paro was emblematic of just the kind of "care robot" *(kaigo robotto)* that I planned to study in Japan, and earliest contacts in the field all referred me to him. When we finally met, I told him about my interest in studying the use of care robots among older adults in Japan. He expressed support and said that he would be happy to provide referrals, but he cautioned that there were only a few nursing homes in Japan where Paro was regularly used. Instead, he told me, the vast majority of Paro sold in Japan were purchased by individual users for use as electronic pets. When I asked him if he could refer me to some of these users, he demurred, citing privacy concerns.

Instead, Dr. Shibata shifted the conversation quickly to the use of Paro in Denmark. A pilot project headed by an enterprising nurse in Copenhagen had concluded the previous year. The project tested Paro's utility in the care of older adults with dementia. The success of the project persuaded the Danish government to order approximately one hundred Paro robots for nursing homes throughout the country. Shibata had recently returned from a visit and had witnessed firsthand how enthusiastically Paro had been taken up. He urged me to go see for myself.

I continued my work in Japan but I would take his advice.

————

Otherwise.

Run Jenny Run.

A few months before the Muratas and I had our meal together, Thomas Schildhauer, a trauma surgeon at Bergmannsheil Hospital in Germany, attended a meeting in Düsseldorf with the Japanese roboticist Yoshiyuki Sankai. Prof. Sankai is faculty in the Graduate School of Systems and Information Engineering at the University of Tsukuba and inventor of the exoskeleton HAL, the very device that I had described to Minoru. As he had on many other occasions, Sankai demonstrated how the sophisticated hardware and software undergirding the exoskeleton worked. Interspersed among the many slides detailing how the mechanical and electrical systems interact within the machine—a system philosophy Sankai calls "cybernics"—were demonstrations of the exoskeleton performed by one of his young, able-bodied assistants. Wearing the HAL suit on his lower body, the assistant strode across the stage without any visible encumbrance; to the contrary, the demonstration climaxed with the assistant lifting a pile of heavy weights without straining. The demonstration drove home Sankai's point: his device could not only help people with disabilities walk independently but could also ease the physical strain of caring for the aged or physically impaired. The demand for such a device would only increase, Sankai added, as the world continued to age rapidly. This was a problem felt acutely both in Germany and in the most aged society on the planet, his home of Japan.

Sankai's presentation was met with general skepticism. Most of the assembled bureaucrats and business managers doubted whether his machine could work in Germany. Dr. Schildhauer, however, thought otherwise. In his hospital work, he operated on patients with traumatic spinal cord injuries and oversaw their programs of post-surgery rehabilitation. He had found that getting a person to move a limb as much as possible, and as quickly as possible, after surgery helped that person recover the greatest amount of function. Might it not be worth trying out the HAL suit in the rehabilitative care of spinal cord injury patients who had recently undergone surgery?

The doctor approached Sankai after he had concluded his presentation and told him about his idea. Intrigued, Sankai invited the doctor to present his ideas at an international research conference in Japan the following spring. That presentation led to a pilot project on the use of HAL with spinal cord injury patients in Germany. The success of the pilot project led to an application to European Union authorities to certify HAL as safe for medical use. The granting of this certification led in turn to investment by Cyberdyne, Sankai's venture firm in Japan, in a facility adjacent to Schildhauer's hospital in Germany. The establishment of this facility elicited an additional round of funding from the New Energy and Industrial Technology Development Organization (NEDO), the research and development arm of Japan's Ministry of Economy, Trade, and Industry, as well as a new research trial with HAL in Germany. That research trial required the recruitment of several participants.

One of them was an ebullient young woman, who later sat across a conference table from me, awaiting my questions. About eighteen months before I met her, Jenny had an accident that partially severed her spinal cord. The accident left her paraplegic and unable to walk without crutches. She underwent standard rehabilitative therapy for six months until she heard about the clinical trial with HAL. Jenny told me that she had made significant progress using the HAL exoskeleton and wished to continue working with it. However, the trial had finished and the therapy was not yet covered by the German healthcare system. Aware of these limitations, friends of Jenny organized a social media campaign to raise enough money for her to continue her rehabilitation. Her friends named the campaign Run Jenny Run, an allusion to the internationally successful German film *Run Lola Run* (1998, dir. Thomas Tykwer). Jenny's actual aims were much more modest than this virtual campaign suggests—she didn't believe that she would ever run again. Nevertheless, the initiative garnered enough support that Jenny was able to continue her therapy, at least for the time being. Unless insurance coverage were expanded to cover HAL "training" (as post-rehabilitative care is called in the facility), it was unclear how much longer she and many other patients in Germany would be able to access the robotic exoskeleton from Japan.

———

Each day seems to bring news of another new robot about to arrive in the world. As I began my early work on this book in summer 2019, for example, the website *The Verge* reported that the American company Boston Dynamics planned to launch Spot, a much-heralded quadrupedal robot that moves with close to the agility of a real dog, as a commercial product later in the year (Vincent 2019). That story was posted just hours after an online feature by the magazine *Wired* on a tech start-up engineering robots to deliver food via bike lanes and a *Washington Post* article on Tesla's plans to convert its vehicles into fully autonomous self-driving cars—that is, a robot on wheels—by the end of the year (Davies 2019; Siddiqui 2019). And that was just one day. Extending the search to a week or several months would yield stories on robots that do surgery, robotic drones that surveil the skies, robots that deliver packages by air, robots that vacuum, robots that mow lawns, robots that cook, robots that work in warehouses, robots that harvest crops, robots that work in hospitals, robots that perform music, robots that tumble like gymnasts, among others. Some of these robots are already here; others remain promises for the future. Whether experimental or actual, the dynamism of contemporary robotics has sparked a range of popular writing on robots and automation, prompting one scholar to claim that we are living in a "robotic moment."[2]

What does it mean to live in a robotic moment? For some, it means that the times are exciting, filled with the expectation that intelligent machines might help make our lives easier. For others, the moment is charged with fear. Robots, and their increasingly "smart" digital cousins, might grow so powerful that they wrest control from their creators to become malevolent overlords, enslaving humans in the way that humans once controlled them. For still others, robotics technologies imperil the economic security of workers, threatening to automate jobs away at a faster pace than new ones are created for those who are displaced. The robotic moment, then, seems to be as much about the future of humanity as it is about the role of machines in the present.

This has been true of robots, in fact, since the moment of their creation. The term *robot* first appeared in the play *R.U.R. (Rossum's Universal Robots)* written by the Czech playwright Karel Čapek in 1920. In Čapek's play, robots are not the jumble of sensors, chips, motors, and metal with which we are most familiar today. They are organic beings, artificial humans that lack emotions and are made to work on behalf of their human creators (Čapek 2004). In the play, robots work so efficiently that they ultimately replace human workers entirely, but a production "defect" leads one robot to gain awareness of their collective enslavement. He (the robot is gendered male) leads a worldwide revolt that results in the annihilation of all but a few humans. The vision of productive but ultimately lethal robots in Čapek's play has had a lasting effect on the Western imagination. Robotic moments then and now often both portend futures of leisure and prophesy the end of labor or even humanity itself.

This book, by contrast, explores another robotic moment, one concerned more with the care of humanity than its pursuit of leisure or its extinction.

Around the turn of the millennium, Japanese roboticists began converting technologies developed for factory production into machines for the care of older adults and people with disabilities. Unlike the robots in Čapek's play and today's factories, these robots have been engineered to sense, anticipate, and respond to changes in human affect and intention; they are *feeling machines*, designed to be *felt* and programmed to *feel*. Over the past decade, so-called care robots have moved slowly out of laboratories into everyday practices of care at home and abroad. This movement has been facilitated in part by governments interested in supporting shrinking populations of care workers without adding pressure on already strained welfare resources. But it is not just the fear of fiscal crisis at work. This robotic moment is undergirded by a transformation in imagining the ends of care such that caring for the aged and disabled by/with feeling machines has become for some not only thinkable but desirable. This book examines the implications of this shift for our understandings of care and our evolving relationship with digital technology.

For scholars of Japan, it seems nearly inevitable that this robotic moment would arrive. Japan is a famously "aged society," and has been for a long time. Twenty-eight percent of Japan's population is currently over sixty-five, giving it the largest proportion of elderly of any country in the world (World Bank 2024). Japan also has one of the lowest birthrates among the low-birthrate countries of the Global North. The close relationship between low fertility and high longevity is widely recognized in Japan, so much so that the social issues are collapsed together as the "low fertility, aging society" *(shōshi kōreika shakai)*. The aging society broke into public consciousness in 1989 and has only grown in intensity since then.[3] In fact, a Pew Research survey found in 2014 that a whopping 87 percent of the Japanese public felt that "aging is a problem," the highest of any country surveyed (Pew Research Center 2014). Over all this time, the country has maintained relatively strict limits on immigration. Only recently has the national government signaled greater openness to foreign workers and reduced obstacles to their establishing permanent residency, in the hope of partially alleviating a shortage of workers in an "aging society" (Smith 2019).

Given a predicted increase in the number of seniors, a projected shortfall of care workers, and continued low levels of immigration, when I began a year of fieldwork in 2010 there seemed few options for Japan other than to supplement human labor with new kinds of machines. Such a turn to machines was not without precedent; robots had help "save" the country once before. Industrial robotics took off in Japan after the oil shocks of 1973 slowed the economic boom of the 1960s, encouraging a shift toward the automation of factory work. The number of industrial robots in Japan rose every year from 1975 through the "bubble" period of the 1980s, boosting productivity and helping Japan reemerge as a global economic superpower (Schodt 1988, 115–20). For most of the twentieth century, Japan led the world in applying robotics technology in manufacturing, giving it a wealth of surplus intellectual and physical capital. An association between technological prowess and economic vitality cemented over this time, and many in Japan came to think of their nation as a "robot kingdom" (*robotto taikoku*; see Schodt 1988, 14). So, too, did contemporaneous observers outside Japan. In an edited volume on robotics, two American experts wrote that "the Japanese . . . are now the most advanced in robotics" (Engelberger 1985, 190) and that "in Japan . . . the robot revolution is further advanced than in any other country" (Wolkomir 1985, 233). Japan's leadership in industrial robotics was matched by pathbreaking research on humanoid robotics and, later, in studies of human responses to lifelike androids (Brooks 2002; Frumer 2018a; Robertson 2018, 110–20). By the late 1990s, Japanese companies had pioneered a range of consumer products that built on this technological heritage, including Sony's robot dog AIBO and innovative devices like Tamagotchi that newly engaged with consumers by eliciting affective connections and generating a sense of intimacy (Allison 2006).

Of course, what *seems* inevitable might not actually be so. When I began my fieldwork in Japan, the actual application of robots in eldercare was quite limited. I did meet individuals who were committed to using robots therapeutically among elderly adults with dementia. However, I encountered just as many roboticists who, though keen to share the promising results of short-term field studies, deferred the real-world application of their machines to the future. Demand for their devices, they assured me, would arrive *someday*, a day that would appear with the many older adults of a future "aging society." These deferrals reflected the temporal inequities embedded in contemporary robotics; the sentiments of those who could afford to luxuriate in the anticipation of a technological future and those older adults, like Minoru Murata, who could not.

Still, while some oriented my gaze forward to a future of care robotics, others like Dr. Shibata and Prof. Sankai directed it *elsewhere* to locations where Japanese machines had already been embraced in the present. Shibata's excitement about the adoption of Paro in Denmark made clear early on that Japanese care robots were more than just a local solution for a local problem of population aging. My study needed to move beyond Japan, but the incipient transformation of HAL *otherwise* into a tool for rehabilitation meant that it had to expand in scope, too, to include younger populations coping with traumatic injury. A project that I had expected to focus narrowly on human–robot interaction among older adults in Japan similarly grew otherwise into a study of a globally dispersed roboscape I call "care robotics 1.0."

Studying Care Robotics 1.0

Over nearly a decade, I followed the complicated itineraries of the first feeling machines from Japan—Paro, HAL, and AIBO. I examined their place in therapy for chronic conditions and traumatic injury across a range of sites. In Japan, I followed a group of robot therapists who use Sony's robot dog AIBO in dementia care for older adults in nursing homes, and talked with roboticists, corporate engineers, government officials, and healthcare workers about care robotics in the present and future. In Denmark, I interviewed civil servants and healthcare professionals, and observed how Paro functioned in therapy for nursing home residents with dementia. In Germany, I spoke with doctors, therapists, and patients working with the HAL exoskeleton, and watched how they set about training with the machine. I coupled these observations of and conversations about care robotics with visits to forums, fairs, and local government initiatives connected to care robots. I supplemented ethnography with archival research on how robots figure in plans and projects to address population aging in Japan and beyond.

This multisited fieldwork was motivated primarily by an interest in how care robots worked "in the wild." While scholars in a range of fields had examined care robots in controlled experiments and short-term field trials, I was curious about what happens outside of laboratories and after field trials end.[4] I wondered: How do patients and nursing home residents respond to care robots in everyday encounters? How do care workers choose to use them? How, if at all, do robotics technologies change prevailing approaches to caring for dementia and disability?

In site after site, care workers told me how robots helped them provide better support for people with dementia and physical disabilities. Some felt threatened by the machines initially but later grew enthusiastic once they realized how they could help them better do what they were doing already. These were professionals who understood well the limits of their own clinical efficacy. In the face of incurable disease or permanent injury, they held no expectation of restoring patients to "normal," to life before an accident or the onset of senility. Whether in the care of dementia or disability, they directed their efforts toward improving the everyday, subjective experience of those living with degenerative disease and irresolvable injury, not to extend the length of life itself.

Indeed, the *feelings* of patients emerged clearly as a primary area of concern for care workers whom I met. In nursing homes, staff aimed to reduce as much as possible the feelings of isolation, stress, and anxiety among older adults with dementia. Manipulating the ability of robots like Paro and AIBO to sense shifts in human affect, they conducted sessions of "robot therapy" that attempted to encourage social interaction and foster connection among older adults in institutional care. Sophisticated robots became cute and cuddly platforms through which moments of social engagement proved therapeutic. Robot therapy did not shift the course of neurodegenerative disease. Rather, it intended to ameliorate, if only for a short time, expression of dementia symptoms.

Training sessions with HAL were similarly targeted at subjective experience. The desire of patients to walk better animated sessions that seemed at first glance to focus so much on overcoming physical impairment. In sessions, patients reported moments in which they felt themselves transcend their physical limitations, as the exoskeleton in turn "felt" their will to move. Assemblages of flesh and plastic, of will and exhortation, moved toward objectives established by the desires of the patient. Training succeeded if patients walked farther, faster, and more confidently than before, even if the nature of their underlying injury did not change. The goals of care were recalibrated if they progressed. Training concluded as it began, rooted in the experience of the patient.

Changing the lived experience of illness or injury without curing its underlying causes emerged as a primary objective across the range of therapeutic interventions I observed. Robots were treated as machines to *care with*. Nowhere did they substitute for the human element of care work or for the kind of person-to-person interaction believed to be fundamental to its performance. Discussions with care workers and repeated observation of their practices demonstrated that robots mediated but did not replace existing relations of care. Ironically, by literally *coming between*, they helped tie individual and collective bodies together. I heard little about the ways in which robots had either transformed or forced innovations in care practice. The more they figured in everyday routine, the less they appeared exceptional.

Yet, even though I initially was curious to see what happens when robots move out of controlled experiments and into everyday life, I learned quickly that the urge to experiment never really ends. The individual nature of dementia and disability make it difficult to know what might work from patient to patient or even from moment to moment. Even within well-defined treatment plans, improvisation and experimentation were essential to good care. At the same time, the successful and unsuccessful use of robots by care workers was of crucial importance to robot makers interested in improving their products. Stated otherwise, the subjective experience of patients had both clinical value to care workers and *economic value* to robotics manufacturers. Therapeutic sites became, in effect, sites of pseudo-experimentation, with care work servicing technological innovation. Experimental impulses extended from robot makers to robot users and back again.

The ecology of experimentation provided robot makers with helpful feedback about the success or failure of robotics technologies. Once patients in Germany strapped on the HAL exoskeleton, they were connected in real time to corporate servers in Japan that tracked, logged, and analyzed their every move. For Dr. Shibata and his colleagues in Japan, feedback on Paro arrived through formal seminars with and surveys of care workers in Denmark. The group of robot therapists I followed in Japan converted their activities into articles and presentations consumed by the makers of the robots they used. Robots channeled feedback even in contexts entirely divorced from institutional care. In "robot towns," ordinary Japanese interact with *(fureai)* the same robots that I observed in sites of care. Feedback from these encounters was captured on surveys and communicated back to manufacturers.

In a range of sites, feeling machines set in motion feedback loops that entangled acts of care in processes of experimentation and innovation. Robots were more than mere replacements for a disappearing supply of laborers. They became platforms for the provision of care *and* the creation of surplus value. As I progressed in my fieldwork, it became hard to disentangle the instrumental interest of roboticists in care facilities from more magnanimous claims about the provision of care technologies for needy individuals now and in the future (see chapter 1). Like the imaginary families of Society 5.0, everyone everywhere was "in the loop."

Iterative Engagements: Care and Creation in Perpetual Beta

In this book, I use the term *iterative engagements* to conceptualize the kinds of interactions that entangle the users and the makers of care robots in open-ended processes of transformation. The term appropriates a concept—"iteration"—drawn from the very software processes that make digital machines work. At the most basic level, iteration describes a process by which software follows a specific set of instructions in a loop over and over again until one or more conditions is met. Each repetition of the loop is called an "iteration," and typically each iteration takes the output value of the previous iteration as its starting point. In a more abstract sense, iteration has come to denote an approach to software development by which various workable versions of a particular software application (or app) are created—that is, they are *iterated*—until a minimally viable version is produced.[5] Each iteration is assigned a "x.x" numerical code that both identifies it and indexes its provisionality. It is expected that bugs will be discovered or that the software will crash or fail in some unexpected way even after it is in wide use. But the errors that appear in the course of everyday use do not signal the end of the process or the failure of any one product to work. Rather, they become the basis for producing yet another minimally viable (or is it maximally viable?) iteration. Iterative development, in other words, is a process that *cannot* advance without inputs of data—that is, without relations of *feedback*—from users external to the technical development process. And, practically speaking, iterative development never ceases. It relies on the frequent release and testing of betas, but even "final" versions of software are in fact not final.[6] (Right now, for example, I am typing on version 16.78.3 of Microsoft Word for Mac running on version 14.1.2 of MacOS while occasionally checking information on the internet via version 120.0.6099.109 of the Google Chrome browser.) Software releases remain in a state of *perpetual beta*, provisional until the next iteration (Neff and Stark 2004).

Iterative approaches rose in cultural prominence along with the expansion of the internet in the late 1990s and early 2000s (Bialski 2020; Seaver

2022). They are not reliant on always-on internet connectivity, but the data collection and algorithmic processing that continuous connectivity affords have clearly accelerated feedback and release cycles. They are now identified with a Silicon Valley–style startup culture and form of digital capitalism perhaps best encapsulated by Facebook founder Mark Zuckerberg's original motto: "Move fast and break things."[7] Moving fast emphasizes rapid development and deployment, while breaking things references a fix-it-later attitude regarding errors and operational failure. The emergence of smart devices—digital technologies made more powerful and responsive through internet connectivity—has only extended principles of iterative development into more and more everyday objects. We increasingly live embedded within techno-social processes that depend, in an intentionally recursive way, on the very way we live our lives.

Viewing care robotics 1.0 as a series of iterative engagements brings into clearer relation the looping processes I observed in the field. Flows of feedback between care facilities and corporate sites are integral, not incidental, to the development process. Technologists rely on the manipulation of their products by care workers just as those same care workers seek out innovative technologies to enhance care delivery. This virtuous feedback cycle exists because of the importance placed on subjective experience for both carers and creators. To say, then, that engaging technologies for care in care is iterative is to emphasize the experimental, even playful, nature of these engagements. Just as perfect functionality is deferred in iterative design, so, too, is a return to "normal" function deferred for those coping with the symptoms of dementia and with debilitating physical injury. Makers and users instead strive not for perfection but for the continual *optimization within as yet unknowable limits* of machines in action, bodies in motion, and minds at rest. Such efforts ultimately may not be therapeutically beneficial or technologically feasible. What matters is a future-oriented disposition of pursuit that enrolls humans and machines in encounters of mutual transformation and that views failure optimistically as an opportunity for future innovation. The futures of iterative engagement unfold otherwise, not through the linear chronicity characteristic of "high modern" state planning (Scott 1998) or demographic projections of "aging society," but in spirals advancing incrementally toward an unknown someday, looping back and forth between here and elsewhere.

This book follows the iterative loops of care robotics 1.0. Its lens is necessarily bifocal: while rooted in specific sites, it attends to relations of human and machine that stretch beyond them. These mutually (in)forming relations put the subjective experience of humans-feeling-machines at the center of both care and technological innovation. Yet robotics 1.0, like all technologies embedded in iterative development, is itself provisional. Across its chapters and through its argument, this book shows how care robotics 1.0 is overtaken by a care robotics 2.0—new kinds of robotics technologies for new care needs, machines that anticipate in form and function the ambient smart technologies of Society 5.0. Care robotics 1.0, then, is as much a moment as it is a category. It is a moment that marks the emergence of new machines for care and new ways of caring with machines. The moment began in the first decades of the twenty-first century, a time when the specter of demographic crisis loomed over a robotics industry in Japan encountering a crisis of its own.

Care Metrics, Care Markets, *Kaigo* Robotics

About twenty years ago, anxiety about the future of care coincided with growing concern about the future of the robotics industry. Japan neared the end of a first "lost decade" of economic growth that followed the collapse of the speculative bubble economy in the early 1990s. Issues that had been obscured by steadily advancing prosperity came to the fore: political corruption, corporate and financial mismanagement, legacies of wartime colonialism, rising disparities in wealth, higher levels of economic precocity among youth, and worrisome demographic trends. The faltering of Japan's surging economy was accompanied by a collapse of a different sort; in 1989, Japan's total fertility rate—the average number of children that a woman has over the course of a reproductive lifetime—dropped to its lowest level since 1966, when a sudden drop in birthrates could be blamed on folk beliefs that deemed it an unlucky year to give birth.[8] Fertility rates would continue to decline until they hit a nadir of 1.26 in 2005, and they remain under the replacement rate of 2.1. While the proportion of Japanese over the age of sixty-five remained below even that of the United States until 1991, Japan surpassed both Germany and Italy in 2005 to become the oldest country in the world per capita, a position that it maintains to this day (Thang 2011; World Bank 2024). Although the causes and consequences of low fertility are distinct from those of high longevity, the two social phenomena are often collapsed together discursively in Japan as the "low birthrate, aging society problem" *(shōshi kōreika mondai)*. They have become a lens through which many in Japan see the present and imagine the future of the nation itself. As an expression of collective sentiment, it is hard to overstate its intensity, particularly with regard to the rising number of seniors.

This is not the first time that population has been problematized in Japan. Malthusian concerns about surplus population drove emigration and settler colonialism from the late nineteenth century into the early twentieth century, much as they did the liberalization of abortion access in the years after World War II.[9] Conversely, fear of depopulation at a time when Japan urgently needed bodies for the military led to a pro-natalist push in the last years of the world war.[10] Even so, earlier efforts to address the size and composition of the national population tried either to support or suppress the birth of children. Rapid population aging, by contrast, was unprecedented. This kind of "surplus population" had never existed. Care of the elderly, formerly a task left to families (primarily daughters-in-law), quickly became an issue of pressing national interest. Rising numbers of elderly appeared poised to overwhelm a public health insurance system that had been made virtually free for older adults to access since the early 1970s. By 1993, individuals over age seventy already accounted for about half of all inpatient care, nearly one-third of whom occupied hospital beds for longer than a year (Campbell and Ikegami 2000, 28). Nursing homes might have accommodated some of these individuals but there were not nearly enough available and they remained stigmatized, perhaps unfairly, as the refuge of those without financial means or secure sources of family support (Campbell 2000). Policymakers set about rationalizing the system of eldercare. They built on earlier efforts and ultimately created a new social insurance program, Long-Term Care Insurance *(kaigo hoken)*, that took effect in 2000.

The new Long-Term Care Insurance program (or, LTCI) reflected a trend toward the "socialization of care" in Japan whereby responsibility for eldercare came to be distributed across state and civil society, not just restricted to families.[11] It presented care services as an earned benefit, not as welfare for the unfortunate. The program's neoliberal framing intended to generate new, high-quality, and competitive markets for care by allowing beneficiaries to apply program benefits to both private and public care providers. Moreover, its name introduced into contemporary policy and public consciousness the term *kaigo*, which been used in government circles to refer to eldercare since the 1970s but had yet had to be inscribed in legislation for the welfare of the elderly. The term proved useful. For policymakers, *kaigo* connoted care for age-related or chronic conditions, conveniently threading a line between acute-care services provided by hospitals (administered by the Ministry of Health) and welfare services provided to individuals needing support in daily life (administered by local welfare divisions). New metrics associated with *kaigo*—quality of life (QoL), activities of daily life (ADL), instrumental activities of daily life (IADL)—unsettled older understandings of health and well-being that had previously grounded public health and social welfare. *Kaigo* also carried an air of novelty and innovation, which made it helpful in marketing a new program (Campbell 2000, 90).

It is no accident that Japan's LTCI system was inspired by a similar program that went into effect in Germany only five years earlier. As in Japan, rising longevity and sub-replacement fertility had alarmed lawmakers in Germany worried about unprecedented strain on welfare resources. The two countries were hardly alone. Nearly all affluent nation-states in the Global North were by then aware of the fiscal implications of population aging. While this shift was particularly acute among the affluent countries of the Global North, the scale of the change was global. Indeed, in 2000, the same year Japan's LTCI system went into effect, the number of people worldwide age sixty years or older exceeded the number of children under five for the first time in recorded history (Kleinman and Hall-Clifford 2010, 247).

The LTCI program and accompanying domestic and global demographic trends did not go unnoticed by the robotics industry of Japan, which found itself encountering a potential crisis of its own. For much of the twentieth century, Japan led the world in the application of robots in automobile manufacturing and other industries (Robertson 2018; Schodt 1988). By the start of the twenty-first century, however, experts in the robotics industry observed that demand for industrial robots had started to weaken. Lower levels of demand meant that robot makers would need to find markets outside of industry. They began to look at the potential of applying robots for nonindustrial use in "everyday life" and in "medical care and social welfare." The industry projected that these two sectors would account for a 5.2 trillion yen (approx. $43 billion, in 2001 valuation) market by 2025, which was nearly four times that predicted for industrial applications.[12] Robots would roam free of factories and begin "coexisting" *(kyōson)* with humans—in communities, in places of business, in homes. The needs of people in these places would become the "problems" that a new generation of robotic devices would help solve, much as they had once done for industry.

The issue was that the roboticists did not have a good grasp about what these needs were or how "next-generation" devices might help satisfy them. Over years of steady demand, the makers and users of industrial robots had built up symbiotic relationships whereby these easily reconfigurable machines were tailored to the specific needs of factory owners. These relationships helped ensure the efficiency of assembly lines as well as the safety of humans working in them. But lower demand meant that such relationships would not continue as reliably as before. Instead, the robotics industry had to consider what kinds of devices could be used safely and effectively in environments that were far less predictable than those of factories. It would no longer be sufficient to develop robotics technologies in laboratories that were cut off from the real world. A future of robot–human coexistence required that everyday environments become fields for technological experimentation, platforms for "open" innovation. Roboticists would call for the creation of "robot towns" where people could interact with robots freely and offer feedback, for new kinds of civilian infrastructure and regulatory frameworks to support their devices, for the opening of robot test fields, and for the establishment of new safety and efficacy standards for machines destined for markets at home and abroad. New models of innovation would be developed that eschewed the linearity of feature request and delivery, and instead sought out the feedback of ordinary individuals. Real-world experience interacting with robots would become a vital part of the development process. The future of robotics innovation would, that is, depend on iterative engagement.

For many in government and in the robotics community, the care needs of a projected surfeit of elders presented just the kind of social problem that the surplus capital of industry might solve. By 2001, the Ministry of Economy, Trade, and Industry (METI) recommended the promotion of robots for eldercare. A few years later, METI would convene a Robot Policy Research Group to consider how robots could help mitigate the economic consequences of demographic aging (Wagner 2010, 138–40). In 2005, the World Expo in Aichi Prefecture featured actual prototypes of robots that had been promoted by METI as part of its vision of robots "as part of everyday life," including prototypes from Toyota and Mitsubishi (Šabanović 2014, 343; Kusuda 2006). Perhaps buoyed by what he saw in 2005, the chairman of Yasukawa Electric Corporation, a major manufacturer of industrial robots, published a book entitled *Robots Will Save Japan* the following year, in which he presents next-generation robots as solutions to Japan's aging society. In 2007, then prime minister Abe's cabinet released *Innovation 25,* a techno-futurist vision of Japan in which humanoid robots would help "compensate for [a] declining and aging population" (Robertson 2007). Yet another METI-sponsored policy research group announced (optimistically) in 2009 that robotic devices for elderly care would be ready for market by 2014. That same year would see the conclusion on the national level of a Robot Care Study Group convened by a parliamentary member of the ruling Liberal Democratic Party (Wagner 2010, 139–40) and the start on the local level of a months-long Care Robot Promotion Project organized by the government of Kanagawa Prefecture. This series of plans, projects, and conferences reflect the interest of a number of stakeholders in applying robotics technology to care for greater numbers of elderly. But they signal just as well the lack of clarity about exactly *how* robotics technology might indeed make a contribution to care. While the impetus for applying surplus robotics clearly came from government and industry, the exact nature of this application would nevertheless rely crucially on the experience of clinicians, therapists, and patients.

Roboticists would encounter clinicians and therapists who had themselves become particularly attuned to the subjective experience—that is, to the *feelings*—of the patients they serve. From the middle of the last century on, medical professionals in Japan and elsewhere began to pay increased attention to the experiences of patients who now were living longer, due in large part (and in a measure of circularity) to advances in biomedical treatments and technologies. Clinicians started to ask not what kind of intervention might help patients live but what might help them live *well.* Increasingly, they took "patient subjectivity into . . . assessments of health care and health," an approach to healthcare that the medical historian Mark Sullivan calls "the new subjective medicine" (Sullivan 2003, 1596). The seeds of the new subjective medicine can be traced to 1948 when, in the preamble to its constitution, the World Health Organization defined health as "a state of complete physical, mental, and social well-being and *not merely the absence of disease or infirmity*" (WHO 1948, my emphasis).

In the following decades, new metrics emerged that attempted to measure physical, mental, and social well-being, particularly among older adults and the chronically ill. These quality-of-life metrics did not just standardize the elicitation of patient assessments in clinical encounters, they also helped constitute a new domain for medical intervention. In the treatment of older adults and those with chronic conditions, quality of life metrics provided a way to target and evaluate care when traditional understandings of cure did not apply. By the turn of the millennium, along with continued efforts to extend the quantity of life through medical intervention, improvement in quality of life "had become a standard means of health care evaluation . . . [that] could provide the goal of health care whatever the age, incapacity or illness of the individual patient" (Armstrong et al. 2007, 368).[13]

Metrics index new areas of collective concern. They make new kinds of medicine possible. They can also make new markets for care. Treatments to raise quality of life became reimbursable through healthcare systems, in turn generating new sources of income for doctors, nurses, and other care professionals. Technologies that facilitated the improvement of quality of life become coverable under healthcare schemes, creating new forms of revenue for technology companies. Measures of quality of life or functional health, in other words, assisted in the conversion of subjective health into a source of surplus value, what the anthropologist Joseph Dumit calls "surplus health" (Dumit 2012). Subjective health as surplus health made how a patient *feels*—the feedback effect of treatments or technologies—the grounds for potential markets and profitability. That is to say, metrics of subjective health created the conditions for *care through iterative engagement*.

By the time that Japanese roboticists turned their attention to the care needs of an aging population, the means and ends of care delivery had changed in meaning from even a few decades earlier. The LTCI system built on global recognition of the value of enhancing quality of life and functional health, and made resources available for the long-term care, or *kaigo*, of the aged and people with disabilities. From this perspective, Japan's *kaigo* robots are very much "artifacts with politics" (Winner 1980). They emerged within specific sociopolitical context marked by the politics of demography and the anticipation of the care burden that unprecedented numbers of seniors would bring. Japan may have initiated one of the world's only national long-term care systems, but the value of long-term care was acknowledged by every major health system in the world. Japanese roboticists would come to see their country as standing at the vanguard of an emerging global market for long-term care technologies. They knew that interacting with their machines would need to enhance the quality of life of potential users. They did not know exactly what kind of machines might be needed, how they might accomplish their effects and for which class of users/patients, or even whether any of this could be accomplished safely. What they needed was feedback on machines designed to care through feedback. The stage seemed to be set for the mutually beneficial encounters of robot makes and robot users examined in this book.

Anthropologies of Technology and Care

By highlighting relations of feedback between robots, robot makers, and robot users, I aim to intervene in emerging scholarship on the role of digital technologies in everyday life, particularly in the areas of health and care. Scholarship on the datafication of health has shown how digital technologies meant to improve health and liberate bodies can also give rise to systems of discipline, surveillance, and control based on the algorithmic processing of health information that is continuously gathered.[14] The findings of this work resonate with studies of the impact of digital technologies more broadly, including the harvesting of big data, the algorithmic manipulation of personal data, the psychological impact of dependence on digital devices, and the creation of new forms of exploitative labor.[15] These processes all depend on the kinds of feedback relations that are operative in care robotics, yet robots tend to be absent from scholarly discussions of digital culture and the datafication of health.

This may be because there are relatively few robots operating in the kinds of domestic, commercial, and healthcare spaces that these studies explore. More likely, the omission reflects a legacy understanding of robots as autonomous, bounded objects—understandings that are less and less reflective of how dependent robots are actually becoming on external infrastructure for sensing and processing power. Contemporary robots can be productively understood as ambient material interfaces for powerful, distributed systems of processors and sensors, or as material platforms for social engagement much like chat apps or social media. They can convert technologies of surveillance and control that are typically fixed to built environments into mobile platforms. Viewing robots in this way can make visible how robots actualize processes of value extraction, surveillance, and datafication captured by other studies of digital technologies and smart devices.

Scholarship on robots in care, by contrast, tends to construe them narrowly as potential substitutes for human care workers. The work of the anthropologist Sherry Turkle, from whom I borrow the notion of a "robotic moment," reflects this sensibility. The robotic moment, she writes, signals the "emotional readiness" (Turkle 2011, 9) of people to accept robots as companions, yet she casts doubt on the suggestion that robots could ever be proper companions. The assumption is that the only role a robot could play is assumed to be one of a substitute yet nevertheless deficient human: "One might say that people can pretend to care; *a robot cannot care.* So a robot cannot pretend because it can only pretend" (Turkle 2011, 124). A care robot is even worse than a human pretender—in essence, it will never be human and so is doomed to fail.

Early on in my research, Turkle's beliefs about the futility of care robotics echoed the reactions of colleagues in Japan to my project. Talk of care robots, they suggested, was just hype. Rarely did they see robots in care facilities. Even when care facilities had them, they often went unused, tossed into closets to gather dust. As one senior American social scientist put it to me in 2011, incredulous: "All they [Japanese bureaucrats] talk about is robots for the elderly. They'll never work!" Years later, the anthropologist Jennifer Robertson would write, "Relatively few robots are actually utilized on a regular basis in hospitals or nursing homes, although experimental prototypes . . . are often presented in the media as if they were widely employed" (Robertson 2018, 30). It seems, paradoxically, that care robots are alarming because they are overhyped and no cause for alarm because they will ultimately fail.

Others claim that robots are valuable insofar as they save money for care facilities, relieve labor for care workers, or do what care workers do but for less money. These economic concerns were of great relevance to the individuals whom I met. But, in practice, robots are rarely used in isolation, much in the same way that hospitals and nursing homes have a range of staff members who together care for patients. The assumption that a robot must function like a human but entirely alone and without the support that human care workers regularly receive from colleagues reflects a notion of bounded *human* subjectivity that has been criticized by scholars for decades.[16] In fact, care robots are used around the world alongside manifold other care technologies. They have support staff just like human carers.

Still, it is true that robots are far from omnipresent in Japanese hospitals and nursing homes, even as of this writing. I have already noted the difficulties I encountered early in my fieldwork in Japan, and in chapter 1 I attempt to theorize the gap between hype and reality that I encountered. Even so, right at the time I was hearing about the present and future failure of care robotics in Japan, hundreds of Paro robots were already in use in Danish nursing homes and Prof. Sankai and colleagues were setting their sights on clinical trials with the HAL exoskeleton. The empirical evidence makes a simple assessment of the success or failure of these technologies challenging. Surely, there is more at work than a Japanese predilection for all things robotic or an inherent futility in applying robotics in the care of older adults or others. (And doesn't some degree of hype accompany the appearance of most new technologies?) Indeed, over the years of my research, the increasingly pervasive presence of digital devices in everyday life positively influenced attitudes toward using robots in care.[17] Working with digital technology came to be an expectation rather than a cause for alarm or surprise.

This openness to technological interventions in care recalls recent anthropological efforts to rethink the meaning of care itself. Studies of care typically assume that "caring actions are best or most naturally motivated by caring feelings" (Buch 2015, 279). Based on a study of family care for older adults in Thailand, however, the anthropologist Felicity Aulino argues that care can be productively understood as a kind of ritual practice in which intention matters less than effective action (Aulino 2016). Ritualized action and habitual practice have meaning within a Theravada Buddhist cosmology in Thailand where one's actions ethically supersede one's orientation toward them. Aulino's perspective opens up a way of considering how good care might obtain while bracketing intentionality. Specifically, in the case of care robotics, it obviates questions about whether a machine *can* care since "right [human] intentions" are not essential to acts of good care.

Such a perspective resonates with recent post-humanist work on care and technology in the field of science and technology studies. Annemarie Mol, Ingunn Moser, and Jeannette Pols suggest that the privileging of the "warm" human touch over the "cold" materiality of care technology ought to be reassessed. "Engaging in care," they write, "is not an innate human capacity . . . Caring practice . . . include[s] technologies from thermometers and oxygen masks to laboratory tests and video cameras" (Mol, Moser, and Pols 2010, 14). That is to say, technologies are not at all opposed to care practices; they enable care, supplement it, affirm it, and extend it. But, just the same, the success or failure of technologies depends on people doing the work of care, "willing to adapt their tools to a specific situation while adapting the situation to the tools, on and on, *endlessly tinkering*" (Mol, Moser, and Pols 2010, 15, my emphasis). Conceiving of care as a form of "tinkering with" the social and the technological, as I do particularly in chapter 3, offers a way of rethinking

the practice of care itself as always already experimental, continually adjust-
ing bodies and minds to new situations and new technology. This is to see
care as a *process* dependent on feedback and response, not just a service that
is delivered or provided unidirectionally. Care then becomes an act of "shared
work" that brings about "the emergence of movement, sensations, possibilities and abilities" (Winance 2010, 95). Thinking of care practices in these
ways avoids transactional hierarchies of dependence and independence, of
care worker and care receiver, or of warm touches and cold objects. Instead,
it aligns acts of care with what I have been calling iterative engagements; that
is, as a generative, rather than merely restorative, process that enfolds both
objects and subjects.

Fields, Methods, Disaster

This book is based on translocal (Zhan 2009) field research in Japan, Denmark, and Germany conducted over a period of eight years from 2009–17. On
a preliminary research trip to Japan in the summer of 2009, I met Dr. Shibata,
Prof. Sankai, and several other roboticists in the Kyoto and Osaka region. I
built out from these initial contacts during an additional eleven months of
field research in the Tokyo area from 2010–11. I met with academic roboticists at the University of Tokyo and other regional institutions, interviewed
bureaucrats about national robotics policy, talked with robot engineers working at major Japanese conglomerates, visited the primary distributor of Paro
and HAL in Japan, participated in planning conferences on robot towns,
attended exhibitions of care technologies, and collected archival material on
care robotics. These experiences provided me with valuable contacts and insights into how elites in the robotics community saw the place of care robotics
in Japan and beyond. Working through these elite networks, I was able to
observe the experimental use of Paro and HAL at three nursing homes and
one hospital on multiple occasions.

At the same time, I actively sought out individuals who worked with
care robots but at a somewhat greater remove from robotics manufacturers
and distributors. A few months into my fieldwork I met a robot engineer-
turned-educator whom I call Dr. Matsuda. Dr. Matsuda led a "robot therapy
group" that regularly conducted sessions of robot therapy, which used Paro
and AIBO among other robots, at a nursing home in neighboring Saitama
Prefecture. I discuss this group's activities in detail in chapter 3, but note

here that Dr. Matsuda took an especially keen interest in my research. He asked me to present my findings to his students and colleagues in Japan, and also invited me to participate in a conference that he helped organize in the United States a couple of years later. Over time our relationship evolved into something resembling colleagues more than foreign anthropologist and native interlocutor. On subsequent, shorter-term visits to Japan in 2012, 2014, 2015, and 2017, I made it a point to visit Dr. Matsuda and observe the work of his group. These additional visits gave me opportunities to revisit initial findings while tracking the significant shifts in the group's approach to therapy over time. Beginning in 2014, I also began following the Sagami Robot Town project in Kanagawa Prefecture, just a few hours train ride south of Tokyo. Visits to the Robot Town and interviews with key officials there provide the basis for parts of chapters 1 and 2.

The vision at the heart of the Robot Town that I encountered in 2014 was marked significantly by an event that occurred three years earlier during my extended fieldwork in Japan. On March 11, 2011, Japan experienced one of the worst earthquakes in its history (indeed, in the recorded history of the world). The quake, which measured a staggering magnitude 9.0 on the Richter scale, was followed by deadly tsunami along the northeast coast of Japan, one of which triggered a nuclear meltdown at the Fukushima Dai-ichi plant. The country has arguably not yet recovered fully from the effects of the triple disasters on its society and economy. At the time, the trauma of the quake was felt acutely by those in the robotics community whom I had come to know. Its aftershocks rattled them in a tragically literal way while also disrupting plans and projects that had been long in the making, including my own. I came to Japan intending to study the development of care robotics for a future demographic crisis, but my conversations with interlocutors were increasingly marked by musings about how robots might help resolve the acute crisis unfolding around us. The quick pivot many in the robotics community made toward disaster robotics in the immediate aftermath of the disaster demonstrated to me how much the "aging society" figured as an expedient rhetorical device for an industry interested in proffering its surplus capital as social benefit. The commitment I found was to apply robotics technology to whatever crisis was at hand, rather than to improve the lives of older adults in the future. I discuss these dynamics in greater detail in chapter 1, but the earthquake is a ghostly presence throughout the book. The trauma it induced underlies the rationale for the Sagami Robot Town; the optimistic vision of Society 5.0 is marked by its conspicuous absence.

The effects of March 11 underscore as well the unpredictability inherent in anthropological field research. Fieldwork is not only impacted by events one cannot anticipate; it also unfolds along a path cleared by the contacts that one makes early in the research process. This book is the product of an initial ethnographic entry into care robotics through the world of those who make the machines, not those who use them. At the time, this seemed the only possible way to proceed. The field of care robotics was highly dispersed and decentralized when I first encountered it in Japan. I knew who the key roboticists were but I did not know who was using their machines or where they were being used. Nevertheless, approaching my field research in this way made me aware of the very feedback mechanisms that are at the center of this book and that have received little attention in other social scientific studies of care robotics.

My ethnographic research in Denmark and Germany, by contrast, proceeded in a different manner. While motivated by what I had learned from roboticists in Japan, it was guided by figures quite distant from the robotics community. In Denmark, a consultant at the Danish Technological Institute led me to a network of dementia-care professionals in Copenhagen and nearby towns who regularly use Paro in dementia care. On weeks-long visits to Denmark in 2012, 2013, and 2017, I observed the use of Paro in dementia care at eight nursing homes and interviewed care workers and administrators about their approach to using the robot. In Germany, an email inquiry to a staff member at Cyberdyne Care Robotics (CCR) led to short visits there in summer 2015 and summer 2017. Officials at CCR generously made staff, patients, doctors, and administrators available for interviews, and permitted me to observe therapy sessions with HAL on multiple days. While I am a fluent speaker of Japanese, I do not speak either Danish or German proficiently. My primary interlocutors in both European countries, however, spoke English with near-native proficiency. When needed, they provided interpreters or interpreted themselves. In some cases, interviewees spoke in a mixture of English and Danish or English and German. I recorded all of these interviews and had these recordings checked, retranslated, and transcribed by fluent speakers of both languages once I returned to the United States.

Structure of the Book

The chapters of the book roughly follow the chronology of my fieldwork. The first three center on research in Japan from 2010–14. The following two focus on Japanese care robots in Denmark and Germany, respectively, and on research conducted from 2012–17. The final ethnographic chapter returns to Japan in 2017. In looping outward from Japan and back again, the book's structure mimics its thematic.

Chapter 1 focuses on the rhetorical linkage between the "future as aging society" and the development of robotics technologies to help solve the problems of this future. Chapter 2 explores how roboticists reimagine the world outside the laboratory as a space that might inspire ideas for new kinds of care robotics. Chapter 3 examines the activities of the Robot Therapy Group of Japan, particularly the way its members use robots like AIBO to help moderate the symptoms of dementia among nursing home residents. Chapter 4 travels with the robot Paro in Danish dementia care, where therapists believe it significantly enhances "quality of life," and the role of Denmark in marketing Paro as a care technology. Chapter 5 follows the feedback loops generated through therapeutic interventions with HAL in Germany, as therapists seek incremental improvements in physical mobility and engineers work toward the iterative enhancement of the exoskeleton itself. Chapter 6 considers the multiple meanings of "care robotics 2.0," a class of robotic care devices that address new care needs and anticipate the feeling machines of Society 5.0. Finally, the epilogue reflects on Japanese care robotics and Society 5.0 in light of the global experience of the COVID-19 pandemic.

ONE

Robots for the Future

On a cool day in March 2011, I sat in a conference room on the twentieth floor of a hotel in downtown Osaka, listening to a Japanese professor of regenerative medicine present a vision of the future city. The professor, whom I call Dr. Kagawa, focused his presentation on the place of medical technologies in an urban development project just north of nearby Umeda train station. His presentation was one of a several scheduled for the day on a part of the development known as "RoboCity CoRE" (CoRE is an acronym for Center of Robotic Experiments). The brainchild of a robotics professor at Osaka University, RoboCity CoRE was envisioned as a project that would capitalize on Osaka's copious human capital to stimulate robotics innovation and, in the process, help ease Japan's future demographic pressures. The audience of approximately twenty-five included academics, policymakers, and representatives from some of Japan's largest electronics corporations.

With Japan having one of the lowest fertility rates in the industrialized world and the largest proportion of seniors, many there saw robots, specifically those designed for welfare and domestic purposes, as both an economic and a social boon; the perfect product for older adults and overburdened young caregivers. Accordingly, part of the RoboCity CoRE plan included a medical clinic serving the needs not only of the elderly but also of the residents of the bustling, mixed-use "knowledge-capital zone" in which it would be located. The bulk of Dr. Kagawa's presentation described the sophisticated network of technologies that would connect the clinic seamlessly to all necessary medical, civil, and social support services in a future Osaka.

No sooner had Dr. Kagawa begun to expound on the importance of such a facility than the conference room started to sway gently back and forth. Dr. Kagawa seemed disoriented. "We're moving, aren't we?" he asked. Those of us in the audience looked around and nodded. "I thought I was just feeling dizzy." Finding it hard to stand, he stopped talking altogether and sat down. I made a note of the time: 2:46 p.m. No one spoke at first as the room began to heave deeply from side to side, as if the hotel was being buffeted by heavy winds. At least, I thought that this is what was happening—the room's curtains had been drawn closed in preparation for the day's presentations. "It's an earthquake (*jishin*)," the man sitting in front of me said, "and a pretty long one at that." "Yeah, but it must be quite far away," an engineer from the Kansai Electric Power Company chimed in confidently, "otherwise we would be bouncing up and down." The feeling of imminent danger having subsided, Dr. Kagawa stood to resume his presentation. I added to my notes: EARTHQUAKE.

Many of us continued listening politely, but it was clear that Dr. Kagawa had lost the crowd. Some attendees flipped open cellphones and slipped outside to check on coworkers and family. Others booted up laptops to send email and follow the developing news. Little did we know at the time that we were experiencing the most immediate shockwaves of a powerful earthquake some five hundred miles away, one that would unleash devastating tsunami and plunge Japan into nuclear crisis. In what in hindsight seems embarrassingly at odds with the historical significance of the events unfolding around us, the meeting went on as scheduled while our room continued to sway for the remainder of the afternoon.

I began following the RoboCity CoRE project during a preliminary research visit to Japan in 2009, and it seemed to hold promise as an ideal future field site in which to carry out an ethnographic study on the integration of nonindustrial robots into everyday sites. Had RoboCity CoRE come to fruition, it may have indeed proved to be such a rich setting. But like many of the attempts to engineer and implement robots for the someday of a demographic future, it did not succeed.[1] I have made reference to the planning workshop devoted to it because the confluence of events that day—techno-scientific project for the future, catastrophic destruction in the present—affirmed for me the gap between imagined futures and everyday exigencies that I had observed repeatedly in the course of my research.

During my early fieldwork, I was struck by how often roboticists I met saw the coming of a "low-fertility, aging society" *(shōshikōreika-shakai)* as the driving impetus for their research. This is perhaps not surprising, given the tremendous attention the subject commands in Japanese media and politics. But in the accounts of my interlocutors, the idea of "Japan as an aging society" was far from just a demographic fact. On the one hand, it emerged as an ambivalent sign of the initial success and later failure of the Japanese state to manage its population; one with considerable motive force. On the other, it was believed widely that managing the risks engendered by this slowly unfolding demographic catastrophe would lead to Japan's reemergence as a global economic player in the future.

In this chapter, I think critically about these imaginings of the future, particularly how they informed the research agendas of the roboticists I met. How was it, I ask, that roboticists came to be so interested in retooling their technology for a future of care? In posing this question, I aim to shift attention away from the potential consequence of population aging to consider what this sociotechnical imaginary (Jasanoff and Kim 2015) *does* for roboticists in the present. The "future-as-aging-society" gives roboticists a rationale to continue developing technologies that seem less vital in an era of economic malaise. It is a future made "legible" (Scott 1998) through technologies of demographic projection and risk assessment, one that reduces uncertainty about the future and calls for its technological management at the same time.[2] But legible futures are not the only possible ones, as the disasters of March 11 made frighteningly clear. Commitment to the future-as-aging-society was an expedient choice, I suggest, not an inevitability. It motivated the iteration of existing robotics technology in the direction of care—in some cases, toward the needs of older adults; in other cases, away from them. And, even when frustrated in the present, it compelled roboticists to continue pursuing iterative engagements of care for the sake of the future.

Imaging Robotics for the Aging Society

An example from my fieldwork helps illustrate the presence of the aging society in the minds of Japanese roboticists. I first met Dr. Yamaguchi, a pseudonym for a member of a research institute at Tokyo University, in February of 2011. His institute is devoted primarily to basic research on robotics and information technology but also develops consumer products in cooperation with major Japanese electronics firms. When I asked Dr. Yamaguchi about the mission and activities of this institute, he began his answer by booting up a PowerPoint presentation that opened with a series of slides organized as much to alarm as inform. "By 2055, the population of Japan will decrease by 30 million people," he said. To illustrate the scale of this overall drop in population, he displayed a satellite map of Japan with just a portion of its topography illuminated. This illuminated green mass represented how much the country's population would shrink, a projection of a living population onto a material substrate. "This will have a huge impact," he emphasized. "Think about the labor force—by 2030 the labor force will decline by 11 million." He showed me two pictures of train cars that were meant to represent Tokyo's crowded Yamanote train line. "Think how jammed in commuters are in the morning; packed in, bursting at the seams." The loss of laborers would equal the emptying out of two train cars in an eleven-car train.

Before I could contemplate how wonderful this would be, he was on to the next slide of his presentation. "GDP will also be affected. Basically, when the population decreases, GDP decreases as well." He showed me a chart comparing the GDP of Japan, China, India, the United States, and the European Union in 2005 to projected GDP in 2025. On the one side, current GDP is represented as children, some bigger and some smaller, with Japan as small but not the smallest. On the other side, each country's future GDP is represented as adults, with Japan the smallest of all—stereotypically so, a diminutive *salaryman* dressed in a navy suit talking on a cellphone.

By 2055, Dr. Yamaguchi continued, the proportion of elderly in Japan will rise from 22 to 40 percent. "Shibuya, the epicenter of urban fashion and youth culture in contemporary Tokyo, might become something like an open-air senior citizens center," he said with a laugh. The population of schoolchildren will drop precipitously, more than halving the average number of children in classrooms from forty as recently as 2005 to seventeen in 2055. The strain of these shifts on public finances will be immense. The collective cost of welfare programs like health care and unemployment benefits will swell to 5 trillion yen per year in 2025. "That's more than the entire annual budget of New Zealand. Every YEAR," his voice rising in exasperation. Pressure on welfare services, he added, will be compounded by shifts in household composition and the size of families. Already, the large extended family, long the provider of care and welfare for the old and young (Thang 2011), is being replaced by disconnected, individualized family units. "As of five years ago, single-person households *(hitori-gurashi)* outnumbered those of other types," he noted. "By 2025, their proportion will rise to 35 percent. What's more, the number of elderly living alone will have more than doubled from 2000 to 2025 . . . This represents a tremendous social change."

The narrative thrust and visual presentation of Dr. Yamaguchi's presentation is striking. As I would find, it was hardly unique. I would hear this stark portrayal of a dim Japanese future articulated by other roboticists I met and would watch it delivered through numerous PowerPoint presentations. I first learned about the RoboCity CoRE, for example, in a 2009 meeting with a professor at Osaka University who was instrumental in its conceptualization. Our conversation began with Prof. Sano booting up a PowerPoint presentation about "Next Generation Robotics Technology in Japan and Osaka." I thought that he would immediately show an outline of the RoboCity CoRE vision. However, the presentation opened instead with a slide entitled "Aging Society in Japan," which was followed by another displaying a line chart of the Japanese population from 1950 to 2100. The trendlines were stark: the aggregate population was set to decrease far into the future, with individuals under the age of sixty-four declining the fastest. A second built out the implications. It placed Japan first among all the countries of the world in its proportion of seniors. The message was clear—Japan's demographic aging was a serious problem; the severity of the problem placed Japan alongside but still ahead of other countries in encountering its implications.

The resonance with Dr. Yamaguchi's presentation is unmistakable. Both men envision a future Japan that emerges directly out of demographic trends that are observable in the present. While this could be seen as an achievement, given the decades of wealth creation, high quality, socialized health care, and relative social order that produced it, this is not its valence in these narratives. Here it is a problem to be solved: millions of intimate decisions about reproduction aggregated and converted into trendlines leading inexorably to social decline and fiscal doom. For the male-dominated field of robotics in Japan, the metaphors are meaningfully, if unintentionally, phallocentric. Shrinking regions, swollen budgets, shrunken *salarymen*, disgorged train cars, dwindling fertility, diminished vitality, senescence—one could even add newly coined categories of emasculated Japanese youth, impotent *otaku* and herbivorous men—all gesture as much to failing masculinity as failed social policy (Chen 2012; Galbraith 2019). The inconsistent mishmash of projected end dates (2025, 2030, 2055, 2100)—which ones match up to which problems again?—do not matter. What's important is that the numbers seem staggering; the endpoints satisfyingly far away yet also disturbingly near. The risk of inaction, catastrophic.

These shared visions of demographic disaster converge around a solution: robotics. Prof. Sano summarized it thusly: "Faced with the major challenge of the aging of society, a falling birthrate, and a declining population, Japan has an increasing need to utilize robots in fields like nursing care and welfare." Robots would help balance the "burden of care" that an increasing number of older adults would place on younger generations. He showed another slide depicting how, in 2050, instead of one couple supporting an aging mother (or mother-in-law), a couple *plus a robot assistant* would help balance the burden. Importantly, these robots did not exist *now* but would need to appear *someday*. For him, this demonstrated the need for the RoboCity CoRE, an urban renewal project in the center of Osaka that would be an incubator for the new kinds of robotics technology that the future aging society would demand. For Dr. Yamaguchi, it provided the fundamental rationale for the Information and Robot Technology Research Initiative (IRT), the research institute at the University of Tokyo with which he is affiliated. Throughout our conversation, he demonstrated the myriad ways in which his institute would "help solve the issues *(kadai)* of the aging society through the application of information and robotics technology."

In these and other roboticists' accounts, Japan's aging society turns from a set of statistical projections into something resembling a *pluripotent signifier*. Like pluripotent stem cells in the body that can develop into any kind of functioning cell, the aging society could be appropriated as a suitably alarming future crisis to rationalize all manner of robotics projects in the present. A professor of mechanical engineering at the Tokyo University of Agriculture and Technology demonstrated for me a prototype of a wearable "power suit for agricultural work" that his laboratory was in the process of developing. He explained that the exoskeleton would help an aging agricultural workforce remain productive into the future, especially for physically demanding tasks like harvesting plums, strawberries, and daikon. A roboticist at the Tokyo University of Science invited me to two demonstrations of another wearable exoskeleton technology, a "muscle suit" *(massuru sūtsu)* that provides power to the wearer when air fills its pneumatically activated artificial muscles. In one demonstration, home health aides tried out the suit to see if it would make it easier to lift older adults who need help getting into the bath (Japanese soaking tubs are usually deeper and narrower than their US counterparts); in another, workers at a logistics company took turns lifting heavy bags of rice, in an attempt to mimic the demands of warehouse work. The rationale for each application converged around problems stemming from demographic change. Increasing numbers of older adults would need assistance with everyday health needs, hence the need to support the workers who will perform this labor. Similarly, with fewer young adults available to take jobs as delivery drivers or warehouse workers, companies will increasingly need to support the bodies of older workers with technologies that can help prevent injury.[3] The roboticist explained to me later in an interview that his muscle suit had a range of applications, from supporting manual laborers in their work to assisting older adults and people with disabilities in everyday life.

Furthermore, in a 2009 report on robotics projects funded by NEDO, a project management arm of the Ministry of Trade and Industry, a representative from Subaru explained that the autonomous cleaning robot they had developed would be of particular value in the aging society: "It will be increasingly difficult to attract workers in the future as the pool of laborers decreases as a result of the low-birthrate, aging society. But this is just the kind of pressure that a cleaning robot can help mitigate. Right now, there is no market for it, but there will be" (NEDO Books 2009, 18). In the same report, a roboticist at ALSOK explained the company's development of a mobile security guard robot in similar terms. "As the supply of laborer decreases due to continued low birth rates and population aging, it will become even more vital to reduce the risk to security personnel of social instability and violent crime. For this reason, and in order to improve the conditions of those working in security, our company has pioneered the development of a security robot *(keibi robotto)*" (NEDO Books 2009, 114).

For some companies, the aging society provides a rationale for developing a whole range of consumer products utilizing robotics technology. At a panel convened by the Ministry of Health and Welfare in the fall of 2010, representatives from Panasonic articulated a vision of robotics technologies meant to "overcome [Japan's] super-aged society" *(chōkōreika shakai ni chōsen suru panasonikku no robotto jigyō)*. The plan envisioned robotics products targeted first for hospitals, then care facilities, and finally for homes. These included robotic machines that could help hospitals prepare medication and deliver them in hospitals to nurse stations, as well as an automatic hair-washing robot and a robotic bed that transforms into a fully functional wheelchair. The latter two technologies would save workers in care facilities from having to carry out these tasks while also preventing injuries incurred in moving nursing home residents from beds into wheelchairs (see chapter 6). By utilizing its surplus capital of robotics technology, the company asserts in another slide, Japan can "transform the liability of the super-aged society into an asset." In this regard, the company had global aspirations. What Panasonic and other companies engineer in Japan for its rapidly aging population could be exported abroad to other countries that are entering the era of population aging as well. From the founding of institutes and urban development initiatives, to robotics products of individual academics, to the highly varied products of corporations, the aging society provides a pluripotent rationale and much needed "problem" for the "solution" of robotics technology.

It is not accidental that all of these companies and all of these academic researchers found themselves so interested in demographic aging in Japan. Demographic aging in Japan had already been problematized by politicians and government ministries for decades. The same ministries helped tie that problematic future to robotics innovation by providing grants specifically for the development of robotic devices for the aging society. In early 2010, about a year before I first met Dr. Yamaguchi, an issue of *METI Journal*, a publication of Japan's Ministry of Economy, Trade, and Industry (METI), focused on robotics meant "to make everyday life better." The issue features many of the robots mentioned above—ALSOK's security robot, Panasonic's robotic bed, Subaru's cleaning robot—in addition to a personal mobility robot prototype from Toyota and care robots like Paro and HAL. Its introductory paragraph makes clear that population aging provides the organizing rationale for the diversity of robotics described in the issue; this is a "better everyday life" in the future, not the present.

By 2015, not only are the total population working population expected to have declined, but the first members of baby-boom generation will enter older adulthood, marking the rapid aging of our society. By 2025, care and welfare support services, which are already understaffed, will need double the number of personnel that they employ presently. One potential solution, which has attracted great interest, is developing robots that can help with everyday needs for care and welfare. As these kinds of robots become more commonplace, people will be able to spend more time doing the kinds of value-added jobs that require the distinctive knowledge and ingenuity of humans. (METI 2010, 4)

This is "everyday life" predicated on the very specific needs of a specific characterization of a future Japan and a future economy. What's more, in words that seem to have inspired aspects of the Panasonic vision outlined above, the journal suggests that other countries will have an interest in such robotics technologies since they will face the pressures of their own population pressures in the future, "giving our country the chance to be the world leader of a new industry, one that builds on our unique technological strengths" (METI 2010, 13). With at once global and local implications, the future of economy and industry is at stake. "The issue may be stated in reverse," the 2009 NEDO report asserts. "The failure to develop robots to assist humans in everyday life itself might provoke anxieties about potentially disastrous effects on economy and industry" (NEDO Books 2009, 112). Affects of "anxiety" *(kenen)* and anticipation run through these accounts of worrisome demographic trends, government initiatives, and robotics projects, all responding to or heightening a sense of impending crisis.

But just who is the target of these interventions? The slippage between the robots for a future of care and for the future of industry and economy, in addition to elisions of local and global markets, is conspicuous and seems deliberate. After all, government ministries like METI and administrative agencies like NEDO must couch their grant opportunities in rhetoric grand enough to attract interest, rhetoric that often conflates economic gains with social benefits. Still, lost in these sweeping visions of a someday are the very aging subjects of "the aging society." They appear as an anonymous, faceless mass, as in Dr. Yamaguchi's depiction of youthful Shibuya transformed into an open-air senior citizens center. Heroic stories of individual longevity are reduced to dots on line charts, meaningful only in the aggregate visual effect of a fearsome rising tide. Navigating later life with declining functional health is reduced to its "burdensome" effects on proximate others and, collectively, on the welfare resources of society writ large. In these abstractions, older adults become good to "think with," a serviceable, defensible target for policy and product development. Nevertheless, meeting the actual needs of older adults, certainly in the present but even in the future, can fail to be a priority even for policies or products meant to address the "aging society." If the risk of an "aging society" is about the burden of caring for frail older adults, then preparing for the aging society means helping people who are *not* frail older adults. If loss of functional independence increases the burden of care, then care delivery should extend from older adults to include children and people with disabilities. If an aging society means a shrinking labor pool, then supplementing the physical strength of those who can work or replacing their labor altogether is a worthy policy goal. If population aging threatens the vitality of industry, then redesigning city centers to foster a spirit of innovation is a sensible response to the demands of the future. For the robotics community, the pluripotency of "the aging society" makes it a currently national but eventually global problem that is solvable by a range of robotics solutions, a fraction of which are meant for the aged themselves. Technologies can change in function and purpose yet still "solve" issues related to demographic change.

Even the identity of the same robotics technology can change depending on the purpose for which it is intended. Although I set out to study care robots *(kaigo robotto)* for older adults, the classification of a robot as a care robot was far from stable. The same robot could be categorized as something other than a care robot even when it was still meant for older adults. In the 2010 *METI Journal* issue mentioned above, a two-page feature story on the robot Paro never uses the term *kaigo* (long-term care) to categorize the robot. Instead, it is described as having a "healing" effect *(iyashi)* on older users (METI 2010, 2–3). Similarly, the issue classifies a full-body prototype of the robotic exoskeleton HAL as an "assistive technology" *(seikatsu shien)* that helps "make it possible for older adults and people with disabilities to eat food or to walk" (METI 2010, 10). These are the very same devices that were included in a local initiative in Kanagawa Prefecture the previous year that focused specifically on *kaigo* robots (see chapter 2). Elsewhere I saw Paro classified as a "communication" or "social" robot, HAL considered a potential "medical device" *(iryō-yō HAL)*, and both robots collapsed together under the rubric of "welfare devices" *(fukushi kiki)*. The many contradictions continue: the front cover of the journal issue shows a young man wearing an early, full-body prototype of the HAL exoskeleton and holding three heavy bags of rice. It is difficult to see how this functionality would serve the needs of elderly individual or people with disabilities.

Depending on the program or sponsoring agency, then, the very ontological status of a robot can change. The *METI Journal* issue included Paro and HAL because they had received funding from a NEDO program to develop assistive robotics technologies for everyday use. Other projects explored the potential applications of robots for medical purposes and welfare applications, and the classification of the robot shifted accordingly. Robot makers had to adjust the rationale for their products in order to secure funds for development. Sometimes this included stretching the meaning of the word "robot" itself. In an interview with me in 2017, an engineer who was involved in the design of the HAL exoskeleton lamented the work it took to receive public support for its development.

> I mean it's frustrating to the point of tears to have to deal with all this bureaucracy, just to get funding to develop your technology. Even the choice to call our exoskeleton the HAL "robot suit" *(robotto sūtsu)* early on was political in a way. You see, each ministry has its own keywords that guide the allocation of funds. Unless you emphasize the "robotic" aspects of your device, you won't be able to access funding from projects run by METI. Likewise, unless your device has some clinical application, you're not eligible for funding from the Ministry of Health, Labor, and Welfare (MHLW). Even if your technology has a specific clinical application, programs differ thematically from time to time, which also can constrain funding opportunities.

Feedback between funding opportunities and the classificatory rationale for robots, even the very conceptualization of their operation, nuances thinking about the relationship between imaginations of a future "aging society" and technologies developed in the present ostensibly to meet its demands. Do the many robots featured in METI and NEDO publications exist because they were conceived as solutions for the pressures of an aging society? Or do they exist *because* METI and NEDO helped support a range of robotic solutions for the aging society? The strategic reframing of the HAL exoskeleton suggests that it is the latter at play. The availability of a technology leads its purposing; the technological "solution" exists before the "problem" emerges. In its pluripotency, the aging society assimilates a range of problems solvable by a range of technological solutions, only some of which directly impact the lives of older adults. It moves from being merely a probable future to a motivating force in the present, manifested in funding programs, research agenda, technology projects, even mundane PowerPoint presentations.

The generative power of the future-as-aging-society is, of course, not limited to robotics development, or even to Japan. By the start of my fieldwork in 2010, it had become a way that the United Nations and other global governing organizations imagined the future of global population.[4] Over the preceding decades, midcentury fears of overpopulation had been replaced by alarm over a looming baby bust and population pyramids teetering on inversion, especially in the Global North. Visions of apocalyptic demography filtered down to states in parts of North America, Europe, and Asia, driving anticipatory initiatives like those in Japan. These initiatives in turn encouraged the flow of policy ideas across borders, hastened the formation of committees and conferences to devise responses, accelerated the development of transnational "care chains," and laid the groundwork for the circulation of products and technologies to meet the looming crisis. The work of academics in documenting and analyzing these manifold developments combined with government forecasts to create a compelling "demographic imaginary" (Aulino 2017).[5] Through the demographic imaginary of the aging society, Japan's political and economic elite could recognize themselves as a part of a global phenomenon of population aging while standing nevertheless at its vanguard, linking Japan both spatially and temporally with the wider world. Members of Japan's robotics community maneuvered within this demographic imaginary, shifting technological development in line with changing programmatic objectives. In the process, whether in the world of policy, in the projects of roboticists, or in the halls of academia, a probable future became increasingly naturalized as an inevitable national fate. Political, industrial, and academic interventions meant to respond to the aging society participated simultaneously, if unintentionally, in its naturalization.

The naturalization of the aging society—its conversion from a probable future to an inevitable one—is, I suggest, deeply dependent on specific temporal assumptions embedded within it. Its linearity is of a piece with twentieth-century theories of modernization, demographic transition, and epidemiological transition—all of which derive from even older evolutionary models of social change. These neo-evolutionary models assume that societies progress in a linear fashion through a series of developmental stages: from tradition to modernity; from high birth and death rates to low birth and death rates; from the age of pestilence and famine to the age of degenerative and man-made diseases.[6] The time of these models unfolds in the future much as it does in the present; it does not expand or contract depending on the kind of activity taking place. Hence, not only can the future state of society be known in advance, the smooth passage from the present to the future can be brought about by rational planning in the present (or, conversely, obstructed by failure to plan properly). Conceptualizations of the aging society embody these assumptions about time and social change, charting a gradual move from a present state of society characterized by population equilibrium to a future state of population disequilibrium that skews toward the aged.[7]

The aging society, like the evolutionary models on which it is based, helps make an uncertain future *legible* and subject to rational intervention. In invoking the term legible here, I borrow from the political scientist James Scott's analysis of the optics of state power (Scott 1998). Scott uses this notion of "legibility" to refer to the many ways in which modern states arrange un-organized populations (and the environment) into units more easily identified and managed—that is, more visible and subject to state power. By conduct-ing population surveys, rationalizing land tenure, standardizing languages, measures, and urban design, among other projects, states attempt to convert unwieldy masses into more efficient, better optimized groups on the basis of models and maps they devise. For Scott such models and maps are not just descriptions of the way society is; they are prescriptions for the way society ought to be organized (Scott 1998, 2–3). The modern state's urge "to create a terrain and a population with precisely those standardized characteristics that will be easiest to monitor, count, assess, and manage" is, he suggests fur-ther, the reason for so many of its failures (Scott 1998, 81–82). The state sees what it wants to see, in so doing missing contingencies and complexities that can frustrate even the best-conceived plans.

Setting aside determinations of failure or success, the vision of the future-as-aging-society that manifests in presentations, policy papers, and program reports represents a similar effort at legibility. But where Scott is concerned with the spatial legibility of territory and population, the aging society is gen-erated by optics of the state that cast forward through time.[8] Though with-out precedent, the aging society is a future that is legible, predictable, and potentially controllable, hence subject to rational planning and intervention. While a nevertheless partial vision, it functions like other technologies of risk assessment in "[converting] future uncertainty into concrete, known risks that are manageable possibilities" (Samimian-Darash 2011, 933). As much as it provokes alarm, it compels actions meant at the same time to ease dismay. The felt need to act inspires "solutions" that recursively affirm the reality of a future that seems virtually here. Affirmations flow across space and scale, from the statistical projections of global and national governing entities to the mundane PowerPoint presentations of academics.[9] In its pluripotent virtuality, then, the aging society makes a future amenable to "governing through time" (Samimian-Darash 2011, 931).

Efforts to make the future legible, just like those directed at space, however, are often cripplingly incomplete. As Scott suggests, the state sees what it wants to see, whether across time or space. It can direct attention forward to probable futures for which it intends to prepare, just as it can deflect attention away from potential futures for which preparation is not possible or even undesired. In the Osaka conference room where I sat on March 11, the potential future of a massive earthquake off the coast of northeastern Japan forced itself, violently and without warning, into the present, during a meeting focused squarely on an aged future that would surely come but had yet to arrive. Over subsequent weeks and months, as the crisis at the Fukushima Dai-ichi nuclear plant worsened, the failure of the robotics community in Japan to prepare for this acute crisis became an item of consternation for interlocutors of mine who had been preoccupied with preparations for the aging society. At first, this seemed attributable to their failure to imagine the "unimaginable" *(sōteigai)*; the inability not just to calculate risk—to tame the future into legibility—but to conceive of risk in the first place. Ultimately, though, it became clear that the issue was more than a lack of imagination. The absence of robots for a nuclear crisis gestured more to the ways in which the imagination is channeled by national prerogatives, directed not only to those futures that *can be seen* but away from futures that one ought not to imagine and ought not to prepare for. The absence of robots ready to handle a nuclear crisis, that is, suggests that nuclear crisis was one future scenario for which preparation, even imagination itself, was not an option.

The Future Unforeseen

A little over a week after the RoboCity CoRE workshop, while the crisis at the Fukushima Dai-ichi nuclear power plant was still raging, I met again with Dr. Yamaguchi at his office on the Hongō campus of Tokyo University. I had requested the interview with an aim to learn about aspects of his research we had not covered in our previous meeting, but our conversation turned quickly to recent events. Unprompted, Dr. Yamaguchi asked me, much like almost everyone else I met those days, about my experiences over the past week. Our discussion then shifted to the subject of robotics and the disaster. "Have you seen the news about the robots that are being used at the Fukushima nuclear plant?" he asked. I nodded in the affirmative.

> Right, well then you know that the Ministry of Defenses ordered disaster robots from the American company iRobot so that they could remotely survey the crippled plant and take samples. This struck me as odd. I know that there are researchers involved in designing and making these kinds of robots in Japan, too. We must have some prototypes. Why did we have to go ahead and order robots from the US? This is rather unfortunate (*zannen*), in my opinion.

Indeed, he proceeded to show me an example of one remotely operable Japanese robot that had been developed for use in disasters. I asked why the government had not chosen to use robots like this in the nuclear disaster. Although the Ministry of Land, Infrastructure, Transport, and Tourism had several of these robots, and had used them for cleanup after earthquakes in the past, he said, "They weren't prepared to do so in this type of disaster. Researchers develop robots like this, and then they show policymakers how useful they are, and then those in power say 'that's great,' but don't follow through. In this case, they didn't do what was necessary to prepare for emergencies."

The situation was in fact more complex than Dr. Yamaguchi implied, or perhaps even knew at the time. Roboticists with whom I spoke after meeting with Dr. Yamaguchi, even those who were committed to projects on the aging society, ruefully recalled how Japan had, in fact, started preparing robots for use in disaster areas following the devastating Kobe earthquake in 1995. But, as several news outlets reported in the wake of the Fukushima disaster, the government only briefly funded efforts to engineer robots for use in nuclear power plants after a deadly radiation leak at the Tōkai nuclear plant in 1999, a date that just predates the shift in public and corporate investment in robotics for the aging society (Chino and Yoshida 2011; Sakai 2011; Vastag 2011). As of March 2011, Japan did not have robots that could withstand the intense radiation in the distressed Fukushima reactor (Kawatsuma, Fukushima, and Okada 2012; Nagatani et al. 2013). In fact, a Japanese robot did not enter the plant until June 2011. A rapidly radiation-proofed "Quince" robot, developed by roboticists at Tōhoku University, made six missions inside the plant until its control cable broke, leaving it stuck inside the number two building (Nakata 2012).

The failure of Japan's robots and civil servants to adequately assess the risk of such a disaster came as a shock and profound embarrassment to the roboticists whom I had come to know. The excuses, explanations, and assignments of blame were manifold. In contrast to the United States, with its well-funded Defense Advanced Research Projects Agency (DARPA), they said, Japanese universities typically do not work on projects funded by the Ministry of Defense; Japan is not involved in any military conflicts that warrant technology robust enough to handle explosions and intense radiation, like the American iRobot; and, as Dr. Yamaguchi suggested, Japan had the technology necessary to build such robots but failed to implement it as a result of bureaucratic incompetence.[10]

Regarding the last of these, Dr. Yamaguchi's sentiments evoke a term that circulated widely in the first months of the nuclear crisis: *sōteigai*. The word can be translated variously as "inconceivable," "unforeseeable," or "unimaginable." It connotes an effort to think of possible futures but also hints at the impossibility of imagining them all in advance. Labeling the confluence of events that led to the nuclear disaster as *sōteigai* became the constant refrain of TEPCO executives (Tokyo Electric Power Company, the operating authority of the stricken nuclear plant) and politicians alike (Bestor 2013; Samuels 2013). Failsafes had been put in place in case the plant were struck by a powerful earthquake. Backup generators had been installed in case disaster knocked out the electrical grid. A fifteen-foot seawall had been constructed to prevent inundation by a massive tsunami. That a massive earthquake would cut off power to the plant, while a nearly fifty-foot tsunami flooded backup generators underground, rendering them useless and precipitating a nuclear meltdown, seemed defensibly difficult to anticipate. As a government spokesman commented days after the meltdown begun, "After the earthquake, the tsunami—a unique, unforeseeable *(sōteigai)* event—then washed out the plant's back-up generators, shutting down all cooling and starting the chain of events that would cause the world's first triple meltdown to occur" (Yukio Edano, quoted in Adelstein and McNeil 2011). In their reasoning, government and TEPCO officials present the future-as-nuclear-catastrophe as the very opposite of the future-as-aging-society. This is a future that existing technologies of risk and forecasting could not make legible. Just as the legibility of the aging society has political and economic implications, so does the illegibility of the future-as-nuclear-catastrophe. For TEPCO and its enablers, this meant a reasonable lack of culpability. Since the powerful earthquake and devastating tsunami were "outside the scope of existing data and records, [the nuclear crisis] was unanticipatable and thus an 'act of nature' for which the company (very conveniently so) could not be held accountable" (Fisch n.d., 1).

A report by the Fukushima Nuclear Accident Independent Investigation Commission, a group convened by the National Diet of Japan, would later dispute this reasoning. It concluded that "TEPCO was too quick to cite the tsunami as the cause of the nuclear accident and [to] deny that the earthquake caused any damage" (National Diet of Japan 2012, 17). What's more, claims of the "unimaginable" notwithstanding, the commission found that TEPCO had been aware since 2006 that a total loss of power could result if a tsunami were to breach the seawall and inundate the reactor site, but had taken no action to mitigate this risk (National Diet of Japan 2012, 16). Investigations of the Fukushima disaster demonstrated that critical voices had been silenced or suppressed. An atmosphere of "bureaucratic inertia" set in, which mitigated against attempts to prepare for a future of nuclear crisis (Kitazawa 2015, 131). This was not a future that could not be imagined; this was a future that the state—allied with industry and even local communities—*did not want to see.*

Critics quickly pointed furthermore to a culture of collusion around nuclear energy in Japan. The Japanese press drew attention to the mutually beneficial relationships of corporate leaders and government regulators who looked past industry failings in exchange for direct compensation or comfortable positions in industry after retirement (Samuels 2013). The regulatory capture distinctive of this "nuclear village," as it is known colloquially, was abetted by a decades-long effort by government and industry to persuade the Japanese public that nuclear power was "100 percent safe" (Kitazawa 2015, 121). Belief in this "safety myth" led to a perversely circular logic. Technologies meant to improve the safety of nuclear power plants could not be supported by either industry or government because their existence alone would suggest that nuclear power was not completely safe.[11] Widespread belief in the safety myth and Japan's condition as a country devoid of plentiful energy resources not only contributed to the country's adherence to nuclear energy, even in the face of accidents in Japan and elsewhere, but also undercut the emergence of any effective anti-nuclear movement. The nuclear village, abetted by the safety myth, worked to render the future-as-nuclear-disaster illegible and unimaginable.

As Dr. Yamaguchi suggested to me, roboticists *had* tried to engineer machines for use in case of nuclear disaster as far back as the 1970s (Onishi 2011). While bureaucratic inertia may have stymied these efforts, it arguably worked in the opposite direction for robotics technologies aimed at the aging society. Bureaucratic inertia in support of a future that the state both could and wanted to see helps explain long-lasting support for care robotics even in the face of obstacles to their widespread application (see chapter 2). Futures made legible or illegible, then, have divergent effects on innovation in the present, either encouraging creation or impeding it. Innovating technologies "for the future" requires technologists to navigate the politics of innovation with shrewdness and savvy.

To my surprise, I saw how quickly this could happen when robots originally meant for the aging society were hastily converted into machines to manage the acute crisis of nuclear disaster. In early May, two months after the disaster, a contact at Daiwa House—the company that distributes Paro—invited me to accompany him on a visit to an arena in Kawasaki City serving as a temporary shelter for evacuees fleeing the areas around the nuclear contamination zone. The company had lent four Paro robots to officials at the site, which at this time housed ninety people. They did so in the hope that the robot might provide some comfort to those who had been displaced, especially older adults. The public relations potential of the effort was hard not to see. Indeed, this was an early test of an initiative that would see the company send Paro robots to temporary shelters and nursing homes in three prefectures that had been severely affected by the disaster. This initiative followed a smaller-scale effort launched a month earlier in the Tokyo area by the robot's inventor, Takanori Shibata.

A Daiwa House press release detailing the effort reported on how much residents of nursing homes enjoyed the robot and how much demand there was for it among nursing home managers (Daiwa House Corp n.d.). But this popularity was not yet on display on the afternoon when we visited the temporary shelter. About a dozen evacuees ranging in age from young to old were brought into a small recreation room. Daiwa house staff put out all four Paro for them to interact with. The kids quickly went over the Paro and immediately started petting them and talking to them. Just as quickly, however, they lost interest in the robots and either started running around the room or playing with other toys. None of the older adults approached the robots at all. This seemed mildly embarrassing to the Daiwa House staff who had invited me to observe for the day. "At other shelters, older people are less reluctant," one told me. "When children are around, older adults tend not to engage." A senior manager at the firm told me of the reluctance of officials at shelters closer to the disaster area to accept the robot, even for free. "Once I start explaining to them that it's a furry robot that looks like a baby seal, they say, 'Oh no, thanks. We won't be needing that.' So, I've just started taking them with me." Another employee concurred, "Yes, it's best to bring it with you and show them that people like it." Yet, there we stood with no one save for a couple of children showing interest for more than a few minutes.

Later that year, in November, Cyberdyne unveiled a newly designed prototype version of its HAL exoskeleton for workers decommissioning the Fukushima plant. The company had reengineered the lower-body version of the exoskeleton to support the weight of the protective tungsten vests workers needed to wear near the nuclear site so they wouldn't "[feel] the burden" (Estes 2011). It was not clear whether this exoskeleton would actually be worn by such workers—it was a prototype after all. But at Japan Robot week the following year, Cyberdyne unveiled a new, reinforced iteration of the prototype. This version added a built-in protective shield, a cooling system to prevent heatstroke, and a chest-mounted sensor to monitor the temperature, pulse, and walking speed of the wearer in real time (*New Atlas* 2012). Despite funding from NEDO to support its development, this version of the exoskeleton was never put into actual operation either. Years later, on a trip to the Cyberdyne headquarters in Tsukuba City in September 2017, I saw a version of this 2012 suit on display in the showroom at the company's headquarters. An engineer with the firm guided me on a brief tour of the showroom, which displayed old and new versions of the HAL exoskeleton beside other company memorabilia. I took pictures as we went along, but this suit was the only item I was not permitted to photograph. I complied with the request but asked to confirm that it was the suit the firm had developed for the crisis at Fukushima. "Yes, but it didn't go into production," he replied wearily. "It had no market, *no market.*" His remark stuck with me. The rapid repurposing of existing technology to manage crisis, a task that ultimately ends in failure, reminded me of so many conversations I had with roboticists about making robots for the aging society.

Daiwa House stopped its free rental of Paro to facilities in northeastern Japan two years after it began and Cyberdyne returned to developing other applications of HAL technology after demonstrating its reinforced prototype in 2012. The immediate shock of nuclear disaster had by then begun to slip into the past, but the ongoing task of nuclear decommissioning work spawned the formation in 2013 of a new government-led entity to oversee the creation of robotics technologies robust enough to withstand the pressure of working inside the reactor buildings and handling contaminated waste material. The International Research Institute for Nuclear Decommissioning (IRID) is made up of eighteen Japanese firms and public utilities, including Hitachi, Toshiba, Mitsubishi, and TEPCO, directed by officials at the Japan Atomic Energy Agency and National Institute of Advanced Industrial Science and Technology.[12] Contrary to initial embarrassment about the recruitment of foreign robots to assist in the first weeks of the crisis, the inclusion of "international" in the name of the organization signals its openness to collaborating with global community on the work of decommissioning, even though the institute is resolutely Japan-led. To date, IRID has employed over twenty robots inside reactors at the Fukushima site, with varying levels of success.

One undeniable achievement of the decommissioning initiative, however, has been the creation of infrastructure in which to test experimental technologies for use in decommissioning work that is expected to take until 2051 (Normile 2021). The Naraha Center for Remote Control Technology Development is located about twelve miles from the Fukushima Dai-ichi site and includes a full-scale mock-up test building in which portions of the nuclear facility can be replicated at reduced scale as well as a building housing a stage and giant screen where engineers can travel through a simulation of the reactor buildings in virtual reality. As the cover of the English-language pamphlet proclaims, the Naraha site aims to "Open Up the Future by Remote Control Technology."[13] Remarkably, a future crisis that had been rendered illegible by belief in the safety myth and by the power of the nuclear village is now not only visible in the present but has become both a literal and figurative platform on which to invent yet other technologies for the foreseeable future. (It is unclear whether IRID really intends to engineer technologies to manage a future nuclear crisis. Its remit, after all, is to resolve a crisis in the present that will extend long into the future.)

The rapid yet arguably unsuccessful enlisting of robots for the aging society into the management of the Fukushima crisis and the equally rapid enrollment of the Fukushima crisis into attempts to create robots for a crisis that was never supposed to happen both point to the inextricable linkages between visions of future crisis and technological development in the present. Inextricable as they are, they are nevertheless flexible. Existing technologies can be quickly, if unsuccessfully, repurposed or repackaged in response to shifting visions of the future or sudden catastrophe in the present. In a move equal parts instructive and ironic, researchers at IRID are interested in investigating how robot technology for decommissioning can be repurposed for the care of older adults.[14]

As much as the future may call for the development of new technologies, actual development of technology for the future can only occur when the regulatory, technological, and physical infrastructure of the present allows it to be brought forth. In a circular way, the future requires scaffolding in the present to bring about its realization. Infrastructure, both material and immaterial, is the platform on which the future is created. For IRID, this required the creation of a site where unimaginable disaster could be made both real and manageable. For roboticists interested in creating robots for the aging society, it meant reimagining everyday spaces as sites where the future of care could unfold, a subject to which the next chapter turns.

TWO

Feeling Machines in Robot Towns

Sometime in 2000, roboticists at the Kyushu-based industrial robotics firm Tmsuk began testing a small remote-controlled humanoid robot. The team had run the robot through mobility tests, all of which it passed. They began to think about next steps. What if we were to test the robot on a sidewalk? Wouldn't any successful humanoid robot need to navigate public space as smoothly as it could the laboratory? They took the robot to a busy shopping street near the city center. Controlling it remotely, they had the robot hand out candies to passersby. The scene soon attracted interest. A crowd formed and eventually spilled onto the street, grinding traffic to a halt. The Tmsuk team quickly concluded the experiment and gathered up its robot.

The following day the president of Tmsuk, Mr. Takamoto, got an angry call from the local police station. The officer on the phone expressed irritation at the fact that the company had endangered lives by interfering with traffic. He requested that Mr. Takamoto come in for questioning right away. Mr. Takamoto met with the officer and explained the team's intentions. The officer's countenance lightened. He realized that he had no grounds to charge the company with a violation of traffic law. Existing law only regulated the use of roads and walkways by pedestrians, animals, and motor vehicles; it said nothing about robots. He wondered aloud whether other companies would try similar stunts in the future and speculated about what kinds of legal scenarios might arise. He suggested that Tmsuk repeat their experiment in Tokyo, where established legal precedent tends to be followed nationwide. He added that the company ought to outfit the robot with an expensive designer handbag. That way, should a car hit the robot, the value of the item would compel police to take the incident seriously and determine fault. Mr. Takamoto complimented the officer on his creativity, but respectfully declined, fearing that the company might still be held accountable even with assurances to the contrary.

In an interview, a Waseda University professor of robotics, who heard this story from the Tmsuk president, told me that not long after the Tmsuk experiment the electronics giant Sony did try to test a small humanoid robot on a public sidewalk in Tokyo. That test also ran into regulatory obstacles. The professor mentioned these two incidents in a conference presentation a few weeks after the Sony attempt. Among the attendees were two officials from Kyushu preference who later drew up a plan to designate parts of cities in Kyushu as "special zones" *(tokku)* for robot testing. They asked for the professor's support for their application to the national government. He obliged, and the prefectural application was ultimately approved. In November 2003, the first three special zones for robot testing in Japan opened in Fukuoka City and Kitakyushu City (Weng et al. 2015, 842).

––––––––––

In the professor's account, roboticists are cast as envelope-pushing innovators who want to try out their newfangled machines in the real world but are stymied by adherence to antiquated regulations. As a narrative, it is not unique. Roboticists I met bought into the vision of the future-as-aging-society, but felt that the existing regulatory infrastructure prevented them from delivering machines for it. In 2009, a humanoid robotics researcher at Waseda University expressed skepticism in an interview with me about the viability of these robots in facilities like nursing homes. Without safety standards, insurance coverage, and enforcement mechanisms in place, the liability risks for companies interested in testing their machines, much less commercializing them, were too great. Two engineers at a large Japanese automaker I interviewed a year later echoed these sentiments. While they wanted to developed mobility devices for older adults, they were not yet able to test them in real-world settings. "There needs to be a general consensus on how to deal with the entry of these devices into society," they told me, "especially regarding what legal regulations and safety standards are appropriate." Japanese doctors and nurses I met that same year were interested in exploring the potential of the HAL exoskeleton in care but were concerned that the machine had not yet been certified by authorities as safe or effective. Officials at Daiwa House, the commercial distributor of Paro at the time, told me that the robot's lack of official certification as a care device hampered its widespread adoption in Japan since its considerable cost could not be partially covered by Long-Term Care Insurance benefits. These frustrations led some roboticists, like the makers of Paro and HAL, to pursue opportunities outside Japan (see chapters 4 and 5) where regulatory environments and funding mechanisms were more favorable. In other cases, it encouraged public and private sector efforts to establish special zones throughout the country where robots for the future could be safely and legally tested in the present.

I continued to encounter robot special zones while doing fieldwork on care robotics in Japan. Sometimes these areas were already existing test sites. In others, they were integrated into urban revitalization efforts. They were always clothed in the language of communal living. Special zones in Kyushu were known as "Robot Town Kyushu." In Gifu Prefecture, there were efforts to establish a "Robot Plaza" and "Robot House" (the "house" later came to be known as the "WABOT House" once it became a testing site for Waseda University robotics). In Ibaraki Prefecture, Tsukuba City opened a "Robot Town" project.[1] A proposal for a "RoboCity CoRE" emerged in Osaka City and "Robot Town Sagami" was later established in Kanagawa Prefecture. Invoking the folksy language of towns and cities might have been an attempt to humanize what are resolutely technoscientific projects. However, it does reflect the popular view among roboticists that future communities will be places where robots and humans peacefully coexist. It affirms the conviction as well that testing "in the real world" is vital to the aims of developing robots for such a future. To engineer robots for the future, roboticists did not just want to move laboratory experiments into public space; they wanted to convert public spaces into living laboratories for robotics development. Robot special zones, in other words, reimagine lived communities as platforms for iterative engagement.

In this chapter, I trace the platformization of urban space in two robot town projects, RoboCity CoRE and Robot Town Sagami, that target the creation of robots for the aging society. These projects emerged at different times—RoboCity CoRE in the mid-2000s; Robot Town Sagami in the 2010s—and they differ in how they incorporate the future-as-aging-society. The RoboCity CoRE vision approaches the aging society as one aspect of human–robot coexistence, while Robot Town Sagami aims to create robots to manage the slow crisis of aging and manage the risk of natural disaster. Where they align is in their shared conviction in the generative power of feeling robots *(taiken)* and their utilization of the platform concept as a means to this end. Feeling machines in the present, safely and legally, promises the iterative realization of robots crucial to care in the future.

Toward Robot Special Zones

In the early 2000s, roboticists were not the only group in Japan interested in removing perceived barriers to technological innovation. At the time, Prime Minister Junichiro Koizumi was busy rolling out a neoliberal reform agenda that urged the marketization of activities traditionally carried out by the state. Official special zone policy came out of efforts to shift away from a state-directed model of innovation toward encouraging entrepreneurship on the local level of municipalities and other regional public-private-academic collaborations (Yashiro 2005, 562). By allowing special tax incentives for industry and "easing" *(kanwa)* regulatory constraints in special zones, officials aimed to foster competition within and between municipalities. The government eventually created two categories of special zones, one for local economic revitalization and another oriented to international competitiveness. By 2014, there were forty-eight special zones in operation (Cabinet Office of Japan 2014).

The principles underlying Japanese special zones align with economic zones in other times and places. "Zoning technologies," to use the anthropologist Aihwa Ong's (2006) phrase, emerged in the colonial era when imperial powers designated ports or other areas of colonial outposts free from normal customs duties or tariffs, expediting the transfer of raw materials or finished goods from the periphery to the metropole. These fundamentally extractive enterprises mutated after World War II into export-processing zones (EPZs) established by global governing bodies like the World Bank and United Nations in parts of Asia, Latin America, and the Middle East. EPZs promised a form of export-led industrialization based on the exploitative integration of native, low-wage, and often female labor into global supply chains (Ong

2006, 102–3). Special economic zones (SEZs) arose in the 1980s when China transformed cities like Shenzhen, Zhuhai, and Xiamen into sites for the introduction of experimental market reforms by loosening regulations in force elsewhere in the country (Ong 2006, 104–5). While SEZs share the liberal economic ethos of EPZs, and often depend on the exploitation of low-wage laborers to manufacture goods and provide services for global markets, they also promise upward mobility for locals willing to work within them. They are "places of imagination and aspiration in which people construct and assemble possible future worlds for themselves and others" (Cross 2015, 424–25). As a form of promissory infrastructure (Hetherington 2016), SEZs spatialize speculation and mobilize affects of expectation. By 2018, there were over 3,500 SEZs distributed across 130 countries (Neveling 2018, 2179). While some are heavily guarded enclosures of factories and workers, others leave few tangible marks on the ground, modifying the sweep of regulations more than the built environment (Bach 2011).

Like SEZs elsewhere, robot special zones are spaces of exception; they combine tax breaks and other incentives meant to attract investment with the suspension of some regulations in the interest of minimizing risk to capital. They also foster affects of expectation and aspiration, firmly oriented toward the future. They are similarly rooted in the extraction of value from assemblages of technologies and people. Yet they are not oriented toward producing goods more efficiently or providing services faster. Nor are they spatially bounded areas that close off a class of laborers from more privileged populations. In fact, much of the infrastructure that makes them function remains largely invisible to human eyes. On visits to robot towns in Tsukuba City and Kanagawa Prefecture, I was struck by how hard it was to identify their material impact on the ground. Instead, they were defined more by their *immaterial* dimensions. These included not only adjustments to the regulatory and business environment but also the sensor technologies, communication networks, and digital data flows that make robot towns legible to robotics technologies. Their multilayered immaterial infrastructure converts ordinary communities into platforms for iterative engagements of humans and robots.

Thinking about infrastructure as a platform might seem at odds with contemporary understanding. Currently, platforms are typically identified with social media sites and the mobile operating systems that facilitate on-demand access to them. Such sites and systems exemplify a view of platforms as "digital infrastructures that enable two or more groups to interact . . . *(inter)me-*

diaries that bring together different users" (Srnicek 2017, 43, my emphasis). It is this intermediating role, rather than their digitality alone, that defines platforms as a new kind of media entity. By *inter*mediating, platforms create value through the delivery of services and the collection of data on the interactions the platform affords. Contemporary digital platforms are inconceivable without the software ecosystems to support them. But they are entirely inaccessible without the hardware on which they run.

Indeed, contemporary platforms originate in hardware, not software. In the 1970s, Japanese automakers introduced the platform as one of a series of innovations in automobile production. Rather than treat each car model as its own, they created modular platforms as "the ground, or foundation . . . upon which different bodies could be placed" (Steinberg 2019, 84). The efficiencies provided by the platform approach contributed to Japan's ensuing dominance in the car industry, and the process was quickly copied by manufacturers around the world. Years later, Japanese industry pioneered yet another influential application of the platform. In the 1990s, the Japanese telecom provider NTT Docomo launched i-mode, the world's first mobile internet platform. Docomo phones equipped with i-mode could access services and content otherwise unavailable on the web. I-mode facilitated new forms of interaction and new kinds of commercial transactions. This made possible the monetization of the mobile internet as never before and paved the way for the dominant smartphone platforms of today (Steinberg 2017, 2019).

It is perhaps no surprise, then, that the platform concept runs thematically through Japanese imaginations of robot special zones. In their earliest conceptions, the technical infrastructure of robot towns functions as a common hardware platform for a variety of autonomous robots, making it easier for different robots to navigate the same urban space. It also makes possible a second-order platformization of robot towns as intermediary sites for everyday encounters between robots and humans. In subsequent elaborations, more elements of the robotic—sensing, information processing, communication—are distributed across the built environment. Urban infrastructure becomes increasingly responsive and robots become less autonomous. Robot towns thus prefigure early on the thoroughgoing roboticization of infrastructure in Society 5.0 as well as the platformization of care robots for the elderly and people with disabilities that I explore in the next chapter.

Revisiting RoboCity CoRE

The conception of urban space as a platform for generative encounters of robots and humans underlies RoboCity CoRE, the project planned for central Osaka City that I described briefly in chapter 1. The RoboCity CoRE project was devised in the mid-2000s along with the formal establishment of robot special zones in Kyushu. Like those projects, the RoboCity CoRE vision assumes that nonindustrial applications of robotics technology in the future will bring about a new society of human–robot coexistence. It also assumes that adapting robotics technology for nonindustrial contexts requires the conversion of everyday spaces into sites for robot experimentation. However, unlike other special zones, RoboCity CoRE is not oriented primarily to the reform of regulatory infrastructure to facilitate the testing of robotics technologies in public spaces. Rather, it moves beyond a view of the field as a site for evaluating the viability of existing technologies and places at the center of robotics development human–robot interaction in the field. RoboCity CoRE imagines the city of robots as a living laboratory for feeling machines.

I first learned of the RoboCity CoRE project in summer 2009 when I met Prof. Sano, a roboticist at Osaka University who was centrally involved in its conception. Our conversation began with a series of slides detailing Japan's apocalyptic demography, much like Dr. Yamaguchi's in chapter 1. Japan's future-as-aging society was meant to underscore the importance of the robotics innovations promised by the RoboCity CoRE project. At the heart of this project is an "open laboratory."[2] Prof. Sano described this space to me as a *"platform* for the design and testing of robotics technology as well as their commercialization and mass production." Like proponents of other special zones, Prof. Sano agreed that creating robotics technologies for a society of human–robot coexistence meant that machines had to be tested in public spaces. But, he added, the function of the open laboratory would be to move beyond the traditional view of the laboratory as a closed "incubation" *(inkyubēshon)* space for robotics technologies. Instead, the open laboratory would bring the process of developing robotics technologies into the view of designers, artists, other researchers, business people, and ordinary citizens. Once prototyped, robots would be placed in an adjacent showroom on the "life of the future." In this space, visitors could "experience" *(taiken)* new robotics technologies and have the opportunity to "touch" *(fureru)* and interact with them, in the interest of providing robot researchers and engineers "feedback on new products and technologies" *(seihin to gijutsu ni fīdobakku suru jisshō-jikken no ba)*. This kind of space would work particularly well in Osaka, he added, because it is in the nature of people in Osaka to be straight-forward with their opinions, in contrast to the more reserved residents of Tokyo. Outside the showroom, mobile robots would roam freely through the commercial and residential spaces of the city. He suggested that this would help familiarize people with the appearance of robots in public spaces and provide municipal officials with insight into what kind of robots people like. In his telling, RoboCity CoRE is intended to be a living laboratory in which new ideas, tastes, and products emerge iteratively through direct contact with a community.

Anticipating my reaction, Prof. Sano admitted that the project sounded idealistic. He added that he was already in discussions with municipal and prefectural officials in Osaka about including RoboCity CoRE in a new urban development initiative in central Osaka. This project, too, was intended to be a global hub for the generation of what its planners call "knowledge capital."[3] The project's mixed-use site of offices, shops, restaurants, and condominiums had at its center a "knowledge capital zone." The zone was intended, much like RoboCity CoRE, as a space where encounters of creators and consumers would generate new forms of valuable knowledge capital. He handed me a glossy, English-language promotional brochure that describes this site as a *"platform where dreams become reality* . . . Knowledge Capital facilitates this by encouraging collaboration across domains and mindsets—businesspeople, researchers, and creators targeting common goals—and promoting constant improvement with *feedback* from general users" (KMO n.d., 5, my empha-sis). In imagining urban space as a platform for the generation of new ideas through constant feedback, it became hard to see where the conception of RoboCity CoRE ends and that of the Knowledge Capital Zone begins. But it is perhaps clear why Prof. Sano believed his project aligned with the goals of the urban development project. At the least, the linkage of RoboCity CoRE and the Knowledge Capital Zone project reflects the salience of the platform concept in thinking about how urban sites might encourage innovation, espe-cially with reference to robotics, in early twenty-first-century Japan.

When I returned to Japan in fall 2010 and later in summer 2012 to talk with Prof. Sano about the status of the project, the RoboCity CoRE concept had begun to evolve from a city for robots to the city *as* robot. Our two meetings bookended the beginning and end of a government grant to support workshops on the RoboCity CoRE project with stakeholders in the Osaka region. A report to which he referred during our conversation represents RoboCity as more than just a living laboratory for the creation of robots. RoboCity itself appears as a roboticized "form of life" *(seimeitai toshi)*, one activated by a shadow infrastructure of sensors, terminals, actuators, and processing units. The report explains why the organizers chose to think of RoboCity as a form of life, using both astronomical and biological metaphors. "First, the entire city is joined together by a network of sensors. Much like a space station, it is an environment of ambient, dynamic intelligence that enables both humans and humanoid robots to work together. Second, in the open laboratory, the 'life of the future' showroom, museums, design offices of RoboCity, the continual replacement of the old by the new resembles the everyday dynamism of a metabolic system" *(Seimeitai toshi: robo-shiti kōsō* 2011, 1). RoboCity is presented as a living thing, a dynamic system that entangles humans and robots in cycles of repair and renewal.

The report continues:

Looking back over the past ten years of developments in robotics, one can see the living city *(seimeitai toshi)* emerge. As recently as the 1990s, most humanoid robots had only a rudimentary vocabulary and performed the same movements over and over. Yet, over that same decade, networking technology advanced dramatically. Now, it is no longer unusual to find reliable wireless broadband connections as readily as wired ones. Robots can now connect to internet infrastructure. Internet-enabled robots do not just have the ability to talk or move on their own. Together with sensors installed throughout the built environment, robots can better navigate public spaces and understand the actions of people within them. This makes them better able to provide service in response to real-time needs. Over the next decade, robots and mobile phones will together emerge as new kinds of neurotransmitters *(shinkei dentatsu busshitsu)* and enzymes *(kōso)* within living cities, helping people communicate and move goods from place to place. Just like good cholesterol helps facilitate the circulation of blood through the body, ambient sensor networks will provide the infrastructure for urban space to function smoothly. *(Seimeitai toshi: robo-shiti kōsō* 2011, 3)

An image on one page illustrates how the roboticized city works (figure 2.1). At lower right, two businessmen enter through ticket gates at a train station. A humanoid robot carries several pieces of luggage for one of the businessmen, while another robot attends to a small child nearby who is alone and seems in distress. Above a video monitor next to the turnstiles, a small antenna juts out with small black waves emanating from it. At lower left, several women prepare meals around a kitchen island located in front of two video displays. Three humanoid robots assist them by washing dishes, stirring a pot, and delivering condiments. Two antennae hang down from the ceiling on opposite sides of the monitors and one sits on top of the kitchen island. The upper right corner depicts a scene from a hospital reception area. One humanoid robot pushes a young man in a wheelchair, another helps an older woman walk with a cane, and a third hands an electronic medical card to an older man using a cane, while a female nurse looks on approvingly. One

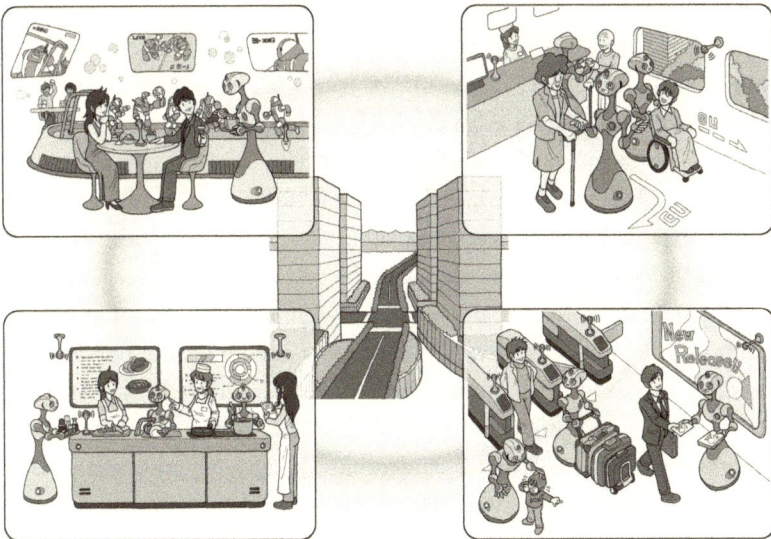

FIGURE 2.1 RoboCity as Living City.   This illustration from a project report on RoboCity CoRE depicts humanoid robots that facilitate the flow of human activity in a city by virtue of their connections to network infrastructure. Source: JST ERATO Asada Project.

antenna is positioned on her desk; another sticks out from the wall. Lastly, at upper left, a humanoid robot waiter visits the table of a couple watching a match of robot soccer.

Although its conception is premised on a future of human–robot coexistence, the proposed RoboCity is not just a place where people passively "coexist" with robots or gather to evaluate them. Robots are thoroughly integrated into the life of the city, actively assisting people as they move through its spaces. They do so by means of their connections to a digital network infrastructure (represented by the many antennae). This sentient infrastructure is a platform that enables robots to provide service and for feedback from human–robot interactions to be tracked. But the organic metaphor of the "living" city suggests something more than simply the harvesting and processing of information. RoboCity takes care of its inhabitants. It is an infrastructure that feels—one that affects and can be affected—populated by feeling machines.[4]

Robot Town Sagami

In 2012, Prof. Sano was confident that RoboCity CoRE would open the following spring. But RoboCity CoRE was never built, despite the completion of the North Umeda Knowledge Capital Zone in 2013. The completed Umeda Zone includes the open laboratory and future life showroom referenced in the RoboCity CoRE project proposal but without robots. As unbuilt and unfinished infrastructure, Robot City CoRE nevertheless provides insight into "multiple visions of the future at play in the past" (Carse and Kneas 2019, 15). RoboCity CoRE conceived an embryonic vision of future robotics in which elements of the robotic are distributed throughout a built environment, thus attending to the infrastructure necessary to introduce robots safely into public spaces. Moreover, it placed public space and public voices at the center of the "open innovation" that a sentient infrastructure helps make possible. This view of roboticized infrastructure would find fuller expression, as well as state support, years later in conceptions of Society 5.0. More immediately in the wake of the RoboCity CoRE failure, the view of robot towns as laboratories for the creation of care robots was realized in a new project established not long after the 2011 triple disasters.

In February 2013, Kanagawa Prefecture launched the Sagami Robot Industry Special Zone *(sagami robotto sangyō tokku)* after receiving approval from the national government. Known colloquially as "Robot Town Sagami," the special zone encompasses the administrative districts of ten cities and two towns that border a major highway bisecting the prefecture on a north–south axis. The stated purpose of Robot Town Sagami is to develop and commercialize assistive robotics *(seikatsu shien robotto)* to "realize the safety and security of local residents" in the future (KLIP 2012, 5). The prefecture's definition of assistive robotics is expansive. It includes not only robots for nursing care *(kaigo robotto)*, medical care *(iryōyō robotto)*, and the support of older adults in everyday life *(kōreisha shien robotto)* but also disaster-assistance robots *(saigai-taiō robotto)*. The pairing of disaster-assistance robots with various kinds of care robotics is the first of its kind but seems an obvious response to the failure of Japanese roboticists to respond adequately to the Fukushima disaster, an experience that would have been fresh in the minds of prefectural residents and officials. While there is precedent for projects linking robotics development with the aging society and for those directed at the development of disaster-assistance robotics, none combines the anticipation of both demographic crisis and natural catastrophe found in Robot Town Sagami.

In the Robot Town Sagami vision, both futures are presented as threats to the "lives"—or, *inochi*—of prefectural residents. The term *inochi* typically refers to life in its biological sense (i.e., the state of being alive) but here it is used in a broad sense to include life *as lived* (i.e., the *quality* of life). It positions robots of the future as technologies that can manage potential disruptions to the reproduction of social life (aging society) or its quotidian rhythms (natural disaster). Even more than Robot City CoRE, Robot Town Sagami frames robotics development as a necessary means of caring for the future. The future needs assistive robotics to support the independence of older adults and to rehabilitate the sick and injured. The future needs assistive robotics because there will not be enough people available to help take care of the older adults who need it. The future needs assistive robotics because disaster may strike suddenly and imperil the lives of rescuers and victims. Humans alone will not be able to support life in the future; more-than-human care is necessary to manage potential crisis, whether it be prolonged (aging society) or acute (natural disaster).

Elements of Robot Town Sagami built on a "Nursing Care Robot Promotion Project" conducted within the prefecture two years before.[5] Like Robot Town Sagami, this project identified the future-as-aging-society as a major threat for which the prefecture needed to prepare. It similarly aimed to stimulate the development of care robots by providing technological assistance for care providers in the prefecture (KWSA 2011, 2). It also made use of care robotics that are featured in Robot Town Sagami. After considering sixty-one potential robotics technologies, the project introduced Paro and the HAL lower-body exoskeleton into four care facilities in the prefecture in order to evaluate their effectiveness.[6] The results were mixed, but the project provided valuable feedback on the kinds of robots that care professionals preferred and on what kinds of obstacles stood in the way of widespread adoption. Much like the feedback process it encourages, Robot Town Sagami iterates on the Promotion Project, broadening its scope to include disaster-support robotics and adopting zoning technology to construct an infrastructure of experimentation and innovation.

The Sagami project offers direct subsidies for research and development (with an initial FY2015 budget of US$6 million), tax incentives, and a variety of regulatory exemptions. It also makes specific locations within the prefecture available as test sites for robot prototypes. The provision of test sites derives from the same interest in getting feedback on robotics technologies found in Robot Town Kyushu and RoboCity CoRE. As the prefecture's application for special zone status notes, it has historically been hard for firms to create assistive robots "because it is difficult to identify what kind of products are needed without opportunities for ordinary consumers to have actual experiences *(taiken)* with them" (KLIP 2012, 15). The special zone is an effort to create the immaterial and material infrastructures necessary to generate the "virtuous cycle of innovation" *(inobēshon no junkan)* (KLIP 2012, 15). This is particularly valuable, a prefectural official in the Labor and Industry section of Kanagawa Prefecture told me, for small- and medium-sized firms. "If you're a big company, you can just build a hospital or similar facility and test your products. This is not the case for smaller firms."

All of these efforts are furthermore directed toward encouraging what the prefecture calls "open innovation," a term which is used differently than in the RoboCity CoRE concept. Here it refers to a process of matching potential consumer demand with a supply of new technologies. The prefecture calls this matching process identifying "needs" and "seeds" *(nīzu to sīzu)*. Open innovation further encourages collaboration among smaller firms with diverse specializations. Rather than struggling to build all technologies necessary for a particular robot, firms are encouraged to share ideas and cooperate creating new products. As much as government recedes from the management of commercial activity by modifying regulatory supervision, in open innovation it actively intervenes by facilitating communication and connection between makers and users.

Robot Town Sagami thus aligns with elements of earlier, failed robot town projects in providing a platform for the open development, testing, and evaluation of robotics technologies. It is doubly charged with affect: it redirects anxiety about future disaster—whether the slow progression of aging or the acute crisis of natural disaster—into the expectation of future innovation. Yet it does so by modifying built infrastructure even less than in robot towns previously envisioned by roboticists. It suggests no new network of GPS devices, RFID tags, or installed sensors. The kind of robots that the prefecture wants to encourage are not those that roam freely in public spaces, as in the RoboCity CoRE vision or even older robot special zones. Rather, the prefecture imagines robots confined to delimited public spaces, such as disaster test zones or tracks of road, or enclosed sites like homes, hospitals, or nursing care facilities. While feedback from the "experiences" of people in such spaces remains vital to the development of future robots, Robot Town Sagami signifies a town of dispersed and delimited interior spaces rather than a dynamic, shared exteriority of public gathering.

Experiencing Robot Town Sagami

The dispersal of open and closed test sites is apparent from the moment one steps within the unmarked boundaries of the special zone. Other than its web presence, there is little of Sagami area's status as a robot town that is observable in its built environment. I found this disorienting when I first visited the special zone, especially given the emphasis on public experimentation in previous plans for robot towns. When I met with an official in charge of administering the zone, he explained that locations in most test sites are used only intermittently by companies and otherwise closed to the public. He suggested that I visit two sites in the zone that are emblematic of its aims and more regularly accessible. The first was an "experience facility" *(robotto taiken shisetsu)*—known by the friendlier nickname "robot house"—and the second a site he called a symbol of the special ward, the Shōnan Robo-care Center. Both sites demonstrate how robot towns reimagine urban space as a

platform for generative interactions of humans and robots. Even more significantly, each encourages visitors to think about the future of robotics through
the lens of care, both the care of others and care of the self.

The Atsugi Robot Experience Facility, one of three such facilities in the
special zone, is located in the heart of Kanagawa Prefecture about a mile
and a half from Hon-atsugi train station. Without a map showing a precise
bird's-eye view of its location, I might not have found it sandwiched among a
dozen model homes on a specially constructed block in the middle of a busy
industrial area. It was not until I stood in front of the property that I saw a
bright red banner bearing the Robot Town Sagami slogan. Visible from a
greater distance were flags advertising the housing firm Daiwa House. As
soon as I stepped inside, it became apparent that the experience facility was
as much an advertisement for Daiwa House homes as a dedicated facility for
the Robot Industry Special Ward.

A representative of Daiwa House met me at the door and welcomed me
inside. Once she opened the sliding door separating the entryway from the
first floor of the house, I could see a hallway that led past a living room toward
a kitchen. Running the length of the hallway on the left side were floor-to-
ceiling stone tiles with one section cut away to make room for a large LED
television. To my right was a framed poster set on an easel that announced the
home as a part of the special zone. Its banner headline read, "Comfortable
(kai-teki): Living with robots is comfortable!" Under the headline was a picture of a three-generation family huddled around a couch. A small humanoid
robot stood next to the couch. "Robots of the future," the text continued,
"will help out with housework and nursing care (kaigo), making your home
life (kurashi) more comfortable." The bottom left corner of the poster depicted
a larger humanoid robot called RIBA carrying a person, next to text reading
"The future will soon be here—Sagami Robot Industry Special Zone."

Past the poster and next to the television was a "HEMS" robot, a device
shaped like a little bird that glows a different color depending on the amount
of energy being consumed in the home. (HEMS is an acronym for Home
Energy Management System.) HEMS aims to give homeowners not only a
visual indication of processes of which they were likely unaware but also to
encourage energy-saving behaviors like turning off one or more devices. The
robot reminded me of large LED screens that displayed real-time levels of
energy consumption that were placed at subway entrances shortly after the
March 11 disaster in order to encourage energy saving. On the kitchen table

was a MySpoon robot arm that helps people with disabilities to eat and drink without human assistance.

My guide led me upstairs into a small, carpeted bedroom, where the lower half of a transparent blow-up doll had been laid on the bed. The doll was wearing a diaper from which two plastic hoses extended down to a large plastic tank next to the bed. The hoses and tank were parts of a care robot called Minelet that detects when a person wearing the device has urinated or defecated, and then flushes the waste material down for chemical treatment in the tank. An explanatory panel explained that this occurs "automatically and hygienically." When the tank is full, a carer, depicted in the accompanying photos as a housewife wearing an apron, can detach it from the device and empty its contents into a toilet. Individuals who are level 4 or 5 on the five-point scale for long-term care insurance coverage are eligible to receive partial coverage for the cost of special diapers and monthly rental of the robot.[7]

I was then led to another room that was furnished like a living room with a loveseat and coffee table. A Paro robot sat on the loveseat with a pacifier-shaped power adapter in its mouth. My guide switched on the Paro robot but did not seem to understand how it worked. Two explanatory panels on either side of the loveseat touted Paro's features and its Guinness World Record as the world's Most Therapeutic Robot. One poster explained how the robot had been developed in response to the limitations of animal therapy, particularly the problems that animals sometimes cause for people with allergies and the difficulties associated with caring for an animal within a nursing care facility. (I discuss this relationship in more detail in chapter 3.) The pictures showed Paro in nursing homes, dementia group homes, and pediatric care facilities, but there was no indication of what Paro might do in a home setting. There was another small doll-like robot on the coffee table called *unazuki-kabochan*. My guide did not know what functions the robot performed. "Does it talk?" I asked. "No, but that one does." She pointed to another room, where a small humanoid robot stood upright on a coffee table. On the diagram of the house, this area was labeled as a children's room.

We entered that room. Past the coffee table, among building blocks and other children's toys, two dolls rested on a faux-wood media cabinet above an iPad, LED television, and Nintendo Wii game console. A poster explained that this was a room for *yasuragi*—or "peace," as the term had been translated into English. "Robots of the future," it read, "will support a peaceful family life. When you feel lonely, they'll be there ready to talk with you.

They'll help you relieve stress *(iyashite kureru)*. They'll adjust lighting, music, even the aroma of a room, to create a soothing atmosphere." At the bottom of the poster was a picture of the same humanoid robot, Palro, that was standing on the coffee table. Palro, the text explains, "talks with people [and] is expected *(kitai sareru)* to help prevent dementia and to reduce the care burden on nursing home staff." I made note of how much work the word *kitai*, or "expectation," was doing in this sentence. Like so many other care robots I saw, Palro's effectiveness was "expected" but yet to be proved.

My guide kneeled down in front of Palro. She switched it on and told the robot to stand up. Palro responded that she needed to unplug it first. She did, and then tried to get it to stand up again. It did not respond. She began paging through the owner's manual for the robot, and asked it to stand up again. Seconds later, Palro stood up and indicated that it was ready to receive further instructions. She leaned close to the robot, operation manual in hand. "Palro, dance! *(odori shite!)*" The robot replied with a loud "Konnichiwa!" and didn't move. "Palro, dance," she implored again. No response. She tried a few more times, perhaps feeling some pressure to make the robot move for her visitor. The robot remained still, like it was stuck in a loop processing the series of commands. All of a sudden, it rotated its arms twice and froze. This appeared to inspire hope. "Palro, dance!" No movement. She flipped through the manual and tried other commands. Nothing happened. "It doesn't seem to be working well today." Resigned, she switched it off.

I asked if the house had drawn a lot of visitors. She said it had attracted great interest when it opened, but that the numbers of visitors had dropped precipitously in recent months. Most visitors tend to be representatives of nursing homes who are interested in seeing what robots can do or "academics like you," she said, smiling. "In fact," she added, "a professor from a local university came just the other day to see what it would be like when robots enter society in the future." Otherwise, she told me, people usually come to look at the house instead of the robots. This made me curious if there were another aspect of the house that buyers would find attractive. She led me to a room about the size of a large walk-in closet with a window overlooking a small backyard on one side and a bench, mirror, and vanity on the other. "This is a space for the wife," she said. Here is where a career woman balancing work and family might get ready for her day. Most houses do not have such a space, she explained, which enhanced its appeal for working families. Intrigued, I asked if there was a similar room for the husband. "No," she replied.

Not every aspect of the experience facility adds up—could two parents really manage working outside the home with both children and a bedridden parent at home? The space nevertheless does express a coherent presentation of technology through affects of care. The robots and material technologies it features are not meant to make the management of home life more efficient or more convenient, as is typically the case in presentations of adjacent smart home technologies. The experience facility works by *feeling* much more than by "thinking." Minelet and MySpoon sense and respond to embodied action, whether intentional or unintentional; Paro and Palro elicit affective engagement through touching and talking. These feeling machines work together with the sustainable yet robust structural materials of the house to generate further feelings of security, comfort, and calm *(anshin, anzen)*. Even energy conservation is assimilated into the rubric of care. Awareness of energy consumption—an affective state facilitated by the HEMS robot—reads as concern for the resources of the Earth. Particularly in the wake of the Fukushima crisis, this extends to the precarious laborers who help convert rare and sometimes dangerous resources into fuel. At the same time, feeling machines in the private space of the home provide technologists with feedback about the functioning of technology in the wider world. Even in its failure to perform during my visit, for example, Palro nevertheless succeeded. Whatever issue caused the malfunction could be addressed. The robot continues to feature prominently in advertisements and events related to the special zone, and still resides in its experience facilities. Such is the logic of the special zone. In making towns and homes platforms for iterative engagement, moments of failure are as informative as moments of success.

Robots for Care of the Self

As much as the robot house facilitates iterative engagements with robotics in the care of the family, the Shōnan RoboCare Center offers a platform for care of the self through feeling machines. The center is located inside a sleek glass-and-steel building in a newly developed district of Fujisawa City, a municipality at the southern end of Kanagawa prefecture in the area of the special zone devoted to assistive robotics for older adults. Shiny hardwood floors and smooth Scandinavian-inspired white surfaces lend it the feel of a high-end fitness club. Three in-floor treadmills might not look out of place, save for the support harnesses hanging over them and the HAL lower-body exoskeletons resting on stands next to them. The only indication that the center is related to the special ward is a poster affixed discreetly in the lower corner of one window with Robot Town Sagami written on it.

The modern look is intentional. My interview with the manager of the center, Mr. Koiwa, reflected the affective atmosphere of expectation that suffuses the center and ties it discursively to the goals of the special ward. "This place is an attempt to offer a new kind of service by applying innovations in robotics technology. That is our 'challenge' *(charenji)*," he told me. At the time of my visit in the summer of 2014, this meant only the HAL lower-body exoskeleton, but he stressed that the center aimed to add additional robots: "Otherwise we would have called ourselves the HAL Care Center." He showed me a rendering of a planned "RoboTerrace" that would double as a showroom for a variety of what he called "useful" *(yaku ni tatsu)* robots, including robots that I had seen at the experience facility (Paro, Palro, Minelet), Segway scooters, and transfer devices to lift people out of bed, among others. The aspiration to provide additional health services with robotics mirrored the intentions of the individuals who came to the center. The version of the HAL lower-body exoskeleton at the center is meant for "general welfare" *(fukushi)* purposes. (In Japan, *fukushi* refers primarily to social services provided by the state to enhance well-being.) In the specific context of the center, Koiwa told me, this meant that the HAL exoskeleton is offered as a technology "that improves life, *quality of life*." People who visit the RoboCare Center seek "care" of this kind. They intend to attach themselves to the robot in an effort to improve everyday functional health and quality of life.

Care *(kea)* at the RoboCare Center, thus, has a specific meaning. The term, a gloss on the English word "care," is written in Japanese using the *katakana* syllabary, lending it exoticism and visual impact. But *kea* has a strategic utility beyond marketing appeal alone. It provides a way of talking about the care of the body in the space between generalized "fitness" and other forms of care that are administratively regulated like nursing care *(kaigo)* and medical care *(iryō)*. As Mr. Koiwa told me, "A device for *fukushi* does not have to produce a measurable effect or therapeutic benefit." At the center, one does not receive nursing or medical care; one *trains*. Although it may look similar to a gym, the point is not to use robots to strengthen one's body for appearance's sake or improve already good health. A person without a physical impairment would not come to the facility. Instead, "training" *(torēningu)* here is directed toward maintaining or improving the functional health of people with a physical impairment of some kind. From this perspective, the center may seem like a rehabilitation center. However, visitors to the center have already been discharged from a hospital or completed a course of rehabilitation but nevertheless have a residual impairment. Since they are no longer under medically supervised care, they cannot apply medical insurance toward the cost of training. (At the time of my visit, HAL was also not officially certified as a medical device.) Since they are not in a nursing care facility or attempting to accomplish a recognized activity of daily life, they cannot apply funds from the LTCI system to pay for their care. (HAL was not an approved nursing-care device either.) Training at the center, thus, takes place within a field of possible health interventions structured by the bureaucratic divisions of the Japanese welfare state.

Mr. Koiwa booted up a laptop to show me a series of slides on the kinds of conditions that people who come to the facility tend to have. Over 70 percent of the people who come to the facility for HAL training have some kind of cerebrovascular disease. Others have a neuromuscular disorder, cerebral palsy, or, in rare cases, a traumatic spinal cord injury.[8] Regardless of their condition, the goals of visitors differ by age. Those in their late seventies and early eighties will likely not see much improvement and, instead, orient their training toward maintaining whatever movement they might have. By contrast, those who are in their thirties or forties orient their training differently. "They anticipate possible improvement and begin training with this goal in mind."

In our conversation, Mr. Koiwa stressed "improvement" over "maintenance." *Kaizen* is a term that has resonance in Japan well beyond the center. For decades, it has been definitive of a Toyotist approach toward maintaining product quality while optimizing the efficiency of production. *Kaizen* relies on workers in all phases of the production process to provide feedback on how best to improve the efficiency of production (Dyer-Witheford 2015, 50). It requires continual surveillance of production processes, since the system can always be better optimized. Hence, *kaizen* is not a *telos*, as ideas like goal-directed or improvement suggest; it is a process that never stops. Accordingly, for a person with a residual functional impairment, this implies continually working toward functional improvement. Importantly, this work stops only when training stops, *not when a condition is cured*. "We don't talk in terms of 'cure,'" Mr. Koiwa stressed. "Otherwise, people would say 'Hey, this isn't a medical device, how can you say that it cures?' Instead, we say 'improvement' *(kaizen)*." If HAL were to be certified as a medical device in Japan, I asked, would you then use the term cure? "No, we never would. We're not a medical facility. We're a *training* facility. A cure would be attempted only in clinical settings under the supervision of a doctor. But, even in that circumstance, working with the HAL suit would be offered as just one of many medical treatments to try."[9]

Touching HAL affords the opportunity to transform the body incrementally. While full physical function may be unattainable, it is not possible either for the wearer or for the staff at the RoboCare Center to know in advance how much functional health might be restored (for younger users) or maintained (for older users). Not only does the technology of HAL afford an opportunity, then, for the delivery of a new kind of care (and a new form of monetizing care), the inherent uncertainty in what might result from care with HAL generates affects of expectation that compel repeated couplings of human and robot. Records of interactions are stored digitally, both by means of the video cameras positioned near treadmills and by virtue of the HAL robot's conversion of user movement into quantitative data. On the basis of this information, users can track changes in physical function just as Cyberdyne examines the strengths and weaknesses of its technology.[10] Although their targets range from individual to family, the RoboCare Center and the experience facility similarly position iterative engagements of human and robot as opportunities for healing. They replicate on the micro-level of interaction the macro-level goal of Robot Town Sagami, inherited from robot town projects before it, to generate future care robots by offering a platform for caring with robots in the present.

————

Compared to several robot town projects that preceded it, Robot Town Sagami has been unusually long-lasting. In 2018, Kanagawa Prefecture launched the second phase of the Robot Town Sagami project. This second phase, which ran until 2022, expanded the kinds of robots eligible for support to include those related to agriculture, forestry, fishing, tourism, construction, transportation, and crime and terrorism prevention.[11] Despite the inclusion of robots that seem only loosely related to the needs of older adults (or disaster assistance), developing robots for the aging society is still the project's organizing frame. The utility of aging society as a pluripotent signifier remains as vital as it did over a decade earlier. Interest in the Robot Town Sagami continues to be robust. A recent annual report on the project details six robotics technologies that were field-tested in the robot town and twenty more that received support for development and commercialization over the 2022 fiscal year.[12]

The sustained relevance of Robot Town Sagami attests to the continued interest of roboticists in getting their machines into the hands of individuals outside of controlled laboratory environments. While this may have stemmed initially from a desire to overcome the risks and regulatory constraints involved in developing robots for purposes other than industry, the elaboration of robot towns over time expresses the equally strong desire to enroll users in the process of technological innovation. Making robots resilient enough to handle operation in dynamic, everyday environments requires insight into how people might respond to machines once they are introduced. It is no longer sufficient to imagine the future of technology in the laboratory alone. Feelings and feedback—the affects of everyday life—become crucial to the future of innovation. But, as the examples of the robot house and the Robo-Care Center demonstrate, feedback is not meant solely to benefit roboticists in the development of technology. Feedback is more than just the fundamental process underlying robotics or the way in which robots navigate public spaces and operate in private ones. It is the means by which machines become technologies of care.

The next chapter explores how a group of roboticists in Japan employ robots in the care of dementia. I suggest that their approach builds on the commitment to feeling and feedback underlying the creation of robot towns. In striving to care with technology, they convert robots into platforms for iterative engagement and transform sites of care into spaces of open experimentation.

THREE

Tinkering with Care

Prof. Matsuda, the leader of a group of robot therapists I studied in Japan, found his way into robotics through a series of accidents. As a child, he was fascinated by planes, space travel, and science fiction. He loved the cartoon character *Astro Boy* and dreamt of one day being an aerospace engineer himself, maybe even building a "real" Astro Boy. Early in 1966, these dreams edged closer to reality when he learned of his acceptance into the engineering program at Waseda University.

On February 5 of that year, roughly two months before young Matsuda would matriculate, an All-Nippon Airways flight was on route to Tokyo's Haneda Airport from Hokkaido when it vanished from radar. Despite reportedly perfect weather conditions, the aircraft had crashed into Tokyo Bay, killing all 133 people onboard.[1] One month later, another plane originating in Hong Kong approached the runway at Haneda after having to circle for an hour in foggy conditions. Its landing gear caught the edge of the airport's seawall, sending it somersaulting down the runway. All but eight of sixty-two passengers perished. Less than twenty-four hours later, a British airliner bound for Hong Kong taxied toward the runway past the still-smoldering wreckage of the flight from Hong Kong. Once airborne, the plane hit severe turbulence, broke apart, and spiraled into the foothills of Mt. Fuji. None of its 113 passengers or eleven crew members survived.

On what *Time* magazine called "the single worst day" in the history of commercial aviation, 180 lives were lost.[2] The accidents undermined public trust in the safety of Japanese aviation. They also shook the confidence of budding young aerospace engineer Matsuda. Could he be responsible for building machines that fired his imagination but could nevertheless so tragically imperil human life? He chose a different path. At Waseda, he switched his course of study to mechanical engineering and entered the laboratory of the legendary roboticist Katō Ichiro.

Katō is well known for his pioneering work in humanoid robotics—his lab would produce the world's first prototype of a functional humanoid robot—but he was also an innovator in the field of prosthetic technology (Frumer 2018b). As a student, Matsuda researched the dynamics of feedback between human beings and mechanical systems, the very kind of systems that had failed catastrophically only a few years earlier. He explored how the faint, myoelectric impulses detectable on the surface of the skin could be harnessed to control the movement of machine limbs and communicate information about their position. By graduation, he had moved on from cyborgian fusions of human limbs and machine parts to examine how image sensors and computer vision could help spot product defects in assembly lines. Interest in automation was high at the time, as Japanese firms attempted to minimize production costs in the face of wildly fluctuating oil prices in the early 1970s (Schodt 1988, 120). His expertise landed him a position in the research and development division of a major Japanese electronics company, where he worked on image processing systems that could identify manufacturing defects in solid-state components, until he hit mandatory retirement *(teinen taishoku)* in his early fifties. After leaving the company, Matsuda took a teaching position in a university department of informatics.

Prof. Matsuda helped establish the Robot Therapy Group *(robotto serapii bukai)* soon after starting at the university. The group, composed primarily of engineering professors and students, visits nursing homes in prefectures bordering the Tokyo metropolitan area to lead sessions of "robot therapy" for older adults with advanced dementia. In sessions, they creatively repurpose robots meant for fun and entertainment into objects of therapeutic engagement. Work with the group returned Prof. Matsuda to an undergraduate interest in the dynamics of feedback between humans and machines. But rather than trying to connect human and machine bodies, the Robot Therapy Group try to generate moments of social interaction among isolated residents using interactive machines. To my knowledge, and despite their lack of specialized training as healthcare workers, there is no other group in Japan that has worked with robots in dementia care for as long as Prof. Matsuda and his colleagues, or in as an intensive and sustained way.

In their aims and methods, one can identify traces of early twenty-first-century calls by robot industry elites to explore the application of robots beyond factory production in such areas as homes and healthcare, especially in light of Japan's "aging society." Indeed, the group's activities align with this interest in appropriating the surplus capital of industrial robotics for nonindustrial purposes. They utilize the capacity of consumer-oriented animaloid robots like Sony's AIBO robot dog and Omron's NeCoRo robot cat, as well as specialized products like the robot seal Paro, to respond to shifts in the affect and intention in order to learn just how best to utilize these very technologies—that is, in a recursive way, to get feedback on the ability of feeling machines to heal through feedback.

Yet, by the time I began to observe their sessions in 2010, the group had long since abandoned the notion that such feeling machines could function alone in the highly unpredictable context of dementia care, especially in individualized human–robot interactions. They learned that they could not treat robots merely as substitutes for human caregiving or for social interaction. Instead, they recognized the need to supplement the real-time operation of their robots with their own intelligence and emotional acuity in group sessions. Caring *with* robots in this manner enables the group to better address their organizing purpose: reducing the psychological stress felt by individuals living in nursing homes, specifically that generated by long periods of isolation and relatively few opportunities for social interaction.[3] To my surprise, this led the team to treat their robots less as machines capable of acting autonomously and more as *de*-roboticized *platforms* for mediated social interaction. In so doing, they preferred "open" robot systems like Sony's AIBO, which permit custom programming and remote manipulation, over "closed" systems like Paro. Open control architectures afford the group opportunities to tinker with, adjust, and optimize the functionality of these robots continually in response to the results of real-world operation. The group came to approach robot therapy as iterative engagement, incrementally modifying technologies and techniques in response to feedback from using robots to care.

In this chapter, I explore the roots of the Robot Therapy Group and analyze their engagement with care robotics. I base this analysis on about a dozen observations of robot therapy sessions during visits to Japan from 2010 to 2017. Given the group's long experience working with robots in nursing homes, I initially expected that these sessions would be strictly routinized. But, as I note above, they turned out to be decidedly experimental. In part this was a response to the challenge of caring for the psychological health of people with dementia—a condition that often leads people to behave in unpredictable ways—with robots that behave perhaps *too* predictably. It was also in part because members of the group are, like Prof. Matsuda, university professors who use this work as grist for their own research and for that of the students with whom they conduct sessions. Fundamentally, I suggest that the group's experimental approach demonstrates an overarching commitment to tinkering with both the techniques and technologies of dementia care in a continuous, iterative way.

These engagements affected both the members of the Robot Therapy Group and their nonhuman companions. For their machines, repeated sessions of robot therapy intensified the "platformization" of robotics technology that I witnessed in initial observations of the group. This platformization happened gradually, as the distribution of control systems across external units and human helpers came to figure more centrally over time. This platformization would be of minor note had it been limited to just the group itself. However, it is emblematic of a broader shift in Japanese care robotics, from the discrete robots of care robotics 1.0 to the distributed robotics of what I call care robotics 2.0 (see chapter 6).

Additionally, for senior leaders of the Robot Therapy Group, engaging robots in care provided a platform on which to construct a reinvigorated, masculine sense of self in the transitional stage of life after the (productive) years of corporate careers end and the (unproductive) years of final retirement begin. Just as robot therapy breathes new life into older robots like AIBO, it gives older members a way to channel surplus vitality and accumulated expertise toward productive ends. Sessions of robot therapy effectively transform the traditionally feminine maintenance work of care into a generative, future-oriented enterprise. Still, the experience of academic and corporate life is not relegated to nostalgia. Prof. Matsuda's time in Katō's laboratory, for example, provided not only a pathway to career but also lifelong connections to a network of influential Japanese roboticists. He drew on this legacy network to acquire the robots and prototypes that made the activities of Robot Therapy Group possible. Even the nursing home where I observed the Robot Therapy Group was run by one of his former classmates. In striving to make the lives of older adults better with care robotics, the aging leaders of the Robot Therapy Group remade themselves as they entered "life 2.0."

From Animal Therapy to Robot Therapy

Prof. Matsuda's life 2.0 in care began in 1999, when he assumed a teaching position at a university in Tochigi Prefecture. Starting a new career after retirement is not unusual for highly educated professionals like Prof. Matsuda. Most large firms in Japan mandate that employees retire in their fifties, and many former salaried workers feel that they still have productive years ahead of them. For Prof. Matsuda, this meant a new, second life in the academy. After teaching in Tochigi Prefecture for five years, he transferred to another university in Tsukuba City, where he worked until 2019 when he would "retire" again, this time for good.

Soon after starting work in Tochigi, Prof. Matsuda happened to see a television news report about a psychiatrist, Dr. Yamaoka, who had started using robots for pediatric care in hospitals. Dr. Yamaoka explained that he had been an enthusiastic advocate of Animal Assisted Activity (AAA) and Animal Assisted Therapy (AAT) before he started working with robots. AAA and AAT are closely related; the former involves interaction with animals and is loosely organized, while the latter uses animals as part of a goal-directed treatment plan. Active, tactile interaction with animals is essential to both AAA and AAT. The intent is to generate feelings of happiness, calm, and comfort through these interactions.

In the course of working with AAA/AAT in hospital care, Dr. Yamaoka later told me in an interview, he began to encounter challenges. The first was feeding. Therapy animals, just like all pets, need to be fed regularly and cared for continuously, which can prove challenging for hospitals that choose to offer animal therapy. Even if hospitals outsource care and feeding, animal therapists still need to secure the approval of the participating hospital and all patients' families. Even if approvals are secured, patients might be scared of animals or have allergies, which limits the population that can engage in such therapy. Furthermore, animals can get stressed or tired through repeated "work" with patients who might unintentionally treat them too roughly. Most surprising to me, Yamaoka encountered what he called "the discriminatory attitude toward animals in Japan." Japanese people, he said, tend to think of animals as "dirty" or "dangerous." This can lead to resistance on the part of some health professionals that borders on the irrational but also manifests in a perhaps more understandable concern that animals might introduce pathogens into an environment where hygiene is paramount.

Frustrated by these limitations, Dr. Yamaoka tried using an AIBO robot dog, a consumer device that had recently been released by Sony, with hospitalized pediatric patients in the same manner that he had previously used animals. Right away, he experienced much less resistance from hospital staff. He learned as well that interactions with robot pets—AIBO to start, later a NeCoRo robot cat released by Omron—provided "stimulation" *(shigeki)* for patients and helped "relax" *(antei saseru)* them in a manner similar to interactions with animals. Using a buzzword of the early 2000s in Japan, Dr. Yamaoka and other members of the Robot Therapy Group described the salutary effect of both animals and robots with the term *iyashi*—a word used popularly to refer to stress relief, relaxation, and restorative feelings of calm. Often this term is used synonymously with the transliterated English word "healing" *(hiiringu)*.[4] This is the kind of "healing" provided by the spas, saunas, or salons that one might visit to relieve the stress of everyday life, rather than to cure a particular ailment or disease. Both robots and animals, Dr. Yamaoka found, helped relieve the anxiety of hospital stays and promote healing-as-*iyashi*.

The news report mentioned that Dr. Yamaoka was scheduled to present at a conference on human-animal relations. Prof. Matsuda quickly registered for the conference and attended the presentation. The two struck up a working relationship and forged a collaboration that continues as of this writing. In 2002, together with interested professors of engineering in the Tokyo area, they founded a Robot Assisted Therapy / Animal Assisted Therapy (RAT/ AAT) Research Group under the auspices of the Society of Instrument and Control Engineers (SICE). The group became a formal chapter of SICE the following year.[5]

The description of the group's mission in its founding documents reflects early twenty-first-century Japanese attitudes toward robotics outlined in preceding chapters. There is the recognition of a "new wave" of robotics technology, one characterized by the arrival of postindustrial "personal robots" *(pāsonaru robotto)* that will coexist with humans outside of factories. This optimistic depiction of inevitable coexistence is followed quickly (though without obvious logical connection) by the recognition that Japan will soon encounter a "super-aged society". In such a social context, personal robots can bring "quality" to the lives of older adults by facilitating "communication" with those around them (RAT/AAT Research Group, 2002). Whereas industrial robots sought to increase the speed and efficiency of production (*quantities* of goods), personal robots instead seek to enhance *feelings* of comfort and satisfaction (*qualities* of experience), a move from the assembly of objects to the manufacture of affects. The pressing needs of this future of aging compelled the group to "pursue the application of robots to the nursing care and welfare [of older adults]" (RAT/AAT Research Group 2002).

Crucially, however, the group's activities would not be limited to care alone. Ultimately, they aimed to turn these affects back into objects. They were interested in exploring the potential of robots for care, to learn about what kinds of robots are most effective, to see what kinds of functionality might be most useful—in short, to discover what value personal robots might bring to society writ large. In language and motivation, the group reflects contemporaneous thinking among elites in the robotics industry who saw everyday life as a new, untapped market opportunity. They recognized early the benefits that robots might bring to sites of care and that sites of care might offer to technological innovation.

AIBO

The vision of personal robots in the group's mission statement is also clearly influenced by contemporary trends in consumer electronics. In late 1990s Japan, a range of electronic products emerged that aimed to provide value for users by fostering relationships of care and nurturance. These products, which the anthropologist Anne Allison has termed "sof-tronics," attempt to cultivate affective bonds with users—ties of "techno-intimacy"—that approximate relations of care between pets and owners (Allison 2006, 188–89). Of course, people have long taken care of material goods. But, in the case of sof-tronic devices, care means more than just treating an object well enough that it stays useful for as long as possible. The very functionality of these devices emerges only through ongoing interaction with a human user. The Tamagotchi, an egg-shaped, plastic toy with an LCD display and three small buttons on the front, is the first and perhaps best example of such a device. When a Tamagotchi is launched for the first time, it gives birth to a virtual pet that is visible to the user via the liquid crystal display. The virtual pet is dependent on the care of its user-owner for its virtual survival. This care is performed by manipulating the buttons on the front of the device to satisfy needs of food, play, cleaning, sleep, and so on. If a consumer does not "care" for his or her Tamagotchi, it will eventually "die" (if only to regenerate again later and start the process all over). Japan's Bandai corporation released Tamagotchi in 1997 and sold forty million within the first year (Allison 2006, 188).

Riding a wave of interest in sof-tronic technologies, Sony released the first iteration of the AIBO robot in 1999. The company marketed AIBO as a "pet-type robot" meant for the entertainment of individual users or families. This was the first attempt by Sony to enter the home market for robotics. Sony intentionally designed AIBO to be small in size (to reduce the risk of injury or damage) and targeted the loose category of "entertainment" where technical glitches would be more readily accepted, even endearing (Fujita 2004, 1804–5).

Key to the Sony AIBO's appeal was the integration of what its makers called "artificial emotions." Based on psychologist Paul Ekman's model of universal emotions, the designers programmed AIBO to express "joy, sadness, anger, disgust, surprise, and fear" (Fujita 2001, 787). Here "emotions" refers to a state of being, more like a mood than an articulation of a specific affect. The robot would respond to human actions differently depending on its mood. When prompted to give a paw while in the state of "joy," for example, the robot dog would gleefully offer its paw. When prompted the same way while in the "angry" state, the robot dog would refuse (Fujita 2001, 785). Artificial emotions operated in combination with artificial "instincts" of hunger, fatigue, and curiosity to simulate more lifelike behavior.[6] Although the device was much more capable than Tamagotchi, it shared the characteristic of emergent sof-tronics in that its very functionality emerged in interaction with one or more human users, making it one of the first feeling machines.

Sony released the first commercial version of AIBO in 1999 and five distinct generations followed until 2003 (see figure 3.1). From the start AIBO was equipped with a range of sensors—including those that could detect touch and sound, measure distance, track movement and position in space—

which gave it the ability to act autonomously in interaction with a physical and social environment. LED lights on its head and back, along with a speaker housed in its chest, provided additional capacity to express emotional states through sound patterns or combinations of colored LEDs. Sony engineers made new combinations of movements and expressions emerge only after users spent a certain amount of time with their AIBO, in a way similar to video games where gamers unlock higher levels of gameplay by progressing through lower-level challenges. This lent the impression that the robot was learning over time much like an actual pet. Sony also made it possible for users to program combinations of movements for their AIBO to perform using a PC-based editor (Sony Corporation 1999). At first, these user-made combinations were saved to a memory stick and then loaded into the robot via a direct connection. By the third iteration of the robot, which debuted in 2001, Sony included a version of AIBO system software that allowed the robot to be controlled via WiFi. Despite some early attempts to regulate how much AIBO "hackers" could adjust system software and access internal data, Sony ultimately released a complete software development kit that let users control nearly all the components of their AIBO for their own noncommercial purposes. Perhaps without intending to, Sony had introduced one of the first software platforms for a consumer robot.

In 2006, Sony stopped manufacturing AIBO and their supply dwindled.

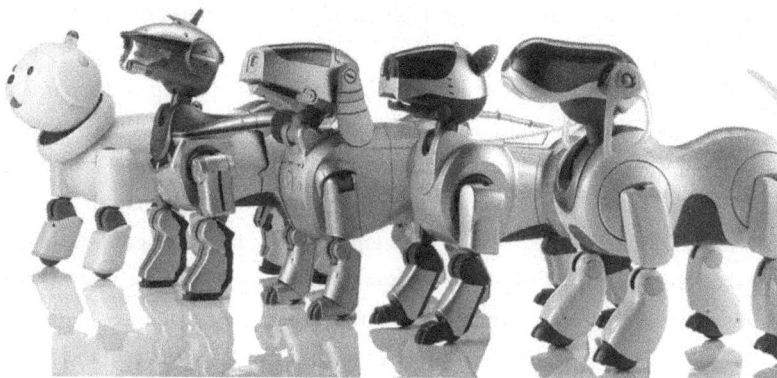

FIGURE 3.1 AIBO Iteration   AIBO models released from 1999 to 2003: (left to right) third generation; fourth generation; first generation; second generation; fifth generation. Used by permission of Sony Electronics Inc. All Rights Reserved.

The robot never proved commercially successful beyond a small group of enthusiasts. Yet, in my conversations with roboticists in Japan only a few years later, it was clear that AIBO had carved out a place of pride among Japanese roboticists. One well-known roboticist I met, who had no affiliation with Sony, bemoaned the company's decision to stop iterating AIBO. "It set Japanese robotics back ten years. There was nothing even comparable to it at the time," he said. I mentioned this comment to an engineer who did work at Sony and was familiar with the AIBO project. While he did not think that AIBO's demise set Japan back, he did agree that Sony's release of AIBO energized Japan's robotics community, providing them with the "courage" *(yūki)* to continue the development of similar products. This technological prowess would be eclipsed in the 2010s by the rise of tech giants like Apple and Google and American robotics companies like iRobot and Boston Dynamics. Indeed, the end of AIBO seems a sign of a broader loss of Japanese status as a leader in technological innovation, especially those for consumers. The Robot Therapy Group continued nevertheless to use multiple generations of AIBO, buying secondhand from enthusiasts who refurbish old models. In so doing, much like Prof. Matsuda and many of the men with whom he worked in the Robot Therapy Group, AIBO was given a second life in care.

Robot Therapy 1.0

When I met Prof. Matsuda and his colleagues in late 2010, the group was in its fifth year doing sessions of robot therapy at Leisure Times, a nursing home in Saitama Prefecture about an hour by train from central Tokyo. Technically speaking, it is a "special nursing home for the aged" *(tokubetsu-yōgo-rōjin-hōmu,* or *tokuyō* for short). *Tokuyō* accept individuals who require the highest level of care under the long-term care insurance system (LTCI), what my Japanese interlocutors describe as the program's "heaviest" *(omoi)* cases. Individuals with relatively "lighter" cases of dementia might be guided to a "group home" *(gurūpu hōmu)* or other healthcare facility. Thus, although *tokuyō* are not specialized dementia-care facilities, nearly all *tokuyō* residents have some form of advanced dementia.

Leisure Times was managed by Prof. Matsuda's friend and former classmate Okada-san. Okada-san worked in Katō's laboratory as an undergraduate student at Waseda University, which is where the two men met, and later went on to a successful career as a systems engineer at a rival electron-

ics conglomerate in Japan. When he reached mandatory retirement around
2002, Okada-san left the company and started volunteering in the front office
at Leisure Times. His wife's family had recently converted farmland they
owned into the nursing home, in anticipation of the new market for such facilities that Japan's recently implemented LTCI program would generate. What
his wife's family had in property they lacked in business acumen. "You might
be able to start a business, but to keep it running over you need somebody
who can think seriously about a business plan," Okada-san told me. His time
volunteering turned into a formal position as manager of the nursing home
where he handles payroll and staffing, among other duties, and even helps out
with nursing care when needed.

Okada-san and Prof. Matsuda stayed in touch over their careers, regularly exchanging customary New Year's cards. When Okada-san learned that
Prof. Matsuda had taken a teaching position in Tsukuba City, he wrote to
tell him that he heard Paro, the baby-seal robot, had just been made available
for sale there. This led to a conversation about Prof. Matsuda's engagement
in robot therapy and subsequently to regular visits of the group to Leisure
Times (now numbering over one hundred and counting).

As a nonprofit, social welfare organization, Leisure Times does not match
the opulence of some for-profit nursing care facilities in Japan. It did, however, look more luxurious than many of the publicly run nursing homes I visited, which tended to resemble Japanese hospitals with their laminate flooring
and numbingly bland concrete walls. By contrast, the main residential space
of Leisure Times is organized in a rectangle surrounding a courtyard with a
small Japanese-style garden and pond. This garden is visible from both floors
through large windows that run the length of the interior hallways. These
hallways are covered in brightly colored carpets that add a cheery ambience
and muffle the sound of shuffling feet. The walls of the facility are filled with
monthly schedules of activities and posters with photos of residents enjoying
recent special events.

Prof. Matsuda invited me to observe several sessions of robot therapy at
Leisure Times in 2010–11. These sessions tended to follow the same pattern.
Members of the group set up their robots in a conference room on the first
floor. They then moved to the second floor, where they pulled several rect-
angular tables together to form two larger square tables. About a dozen residents, all in wheelchairs, were brought into the room by staff and positioned
around the tables. Others, who could still walk well enough, found their own

places. As they came in, Okada-san announced their names in a voice loud enough for everyone to hear. Members answered with a hearty "Konnichiwa!" With the residents seated around the tables, the activity began.

On one particular day I watch as the team places robots on the tables in front of the seated residents, staggering about one robot per two or three residents. The robots include two robot cats (NeCoRo) and several AIBO robot dogs. As soon as the robots are placed on the table, the residents begin to fiddle with them—touching them, petting them, smiling at them, talking to them. Professors and students, who just a moment before had been intensely engaged in preparation, suddenly become amateur entertainers. They circulate among the seated residents, careful to crouch down to their level when talking with them. They help facilitate the residents' verbal and tactile interactions with the robots. They tell them how to get the robots to respond to touch or to voice, serving as prosthetic ears by repeating sounds coming from the robots when residents have trouble hearing them.

Across the room, I see another table with a laptop on it. Two male undergraduates and their professor huddle around it with their eyes fixed on the screen. An AIBO robot is next to the laptop, its head moving in fits and starts. They position the robot upright and it takes a few steps back and forth. As I'm trying to figure out what they are doing, a woman enters the room with her back bent at a nearly ninety-degree angle. One of her arms hangs down in front of her and the other is hidden under the waistband of her pants below her lower back, as if she were trying to tuck in her shirt. The professor and students near the laptop watch her carefully as she finds a seat at one table. A few minutes later, one of the students walks over and places the AIBO robot in front of her. He returns to the table and to the laptop. The professor leaves to join his colleagues but his students keep their eyes on the woman.

In conversations with staff on previous visits to the nursing home, these students learned that the woman habitually roams around the hallways of the nursing home. She would also sing to herself and pound loudly on tables while sitting with other residents, ignoring the instructions of nursing home staff to stop, and occasionally would enter the rooms of other residents uninvited. Roaming as well as these other actions are behavioral symptoms of dementia. Nursing home staff interpreted them as expressions of stress, anxiety, or isolation. The students were curious to see if the frequency of these behaviors would change after one-on-one interactions with the robot. To gauge the effect, the students arrived in advance of the group to record the woman's movements in five-minute intervals. They repeated this protocol after the robot therapy session to measure any changes in the frequency or character of her wandering around the nursing home.[7]

Using the software development platform that Sony had installed, the students worked with their professor to write a program that triggered movements in the AIBO robot on demand. The program also enabled them to activate multicolored LEDs on the robot's body in patterns or to play prerecorded sounds and phrases through the robot's speaker. While Sony originally designed the machine such that these kinds of actions would emerge organically in the course of everyday interaction with a consumer "owner," the cultivation of such intimacy is unrealistic in nursing homes where individual time with robots is limited. Members of the robot therapy team instead supplement the capacity of the robot to sense, respond, and learn with their own.

To choreograph the behavior of the robot, they were aided by the ability of later generations of AIBO to be remotely controlled via WiFi. (They set up a proxy WiFi network in the room to make this possible.) Such direct control was not limited just to this experiment. The professors in the Robot Therapy Group, all of them engineers, favored the open operating system of robots like AIBO over those of robots such as Paro or NeCoRo, which could not be manipulated remotely or reprogrammed by anyone other than the manufacturer. On every one of my visits, there were always at least one or more AIBO robots that were controlled in this way. While the fur covering of a Paro or NeCoRo robot might invite an individual to touch or embrace it, the open architecture of the AIBO robot facilitated collective interaction and engagement. It made possible the real-time orchestration of a form of controlled play that is at once more-than-human and more-than-robotic.

As I watch, the tight control of the student experiment contrasts starkly with the thinly organized chaos unfolding around me. Machines whir and whimper. Songs and sounds blare out. Attention is attracted and then suddenly diverted. Conversations start and are promptly interrupted. Robots run out of juice, suddenly freeze, or get tripped up and fall over with a crash. Members of the group and nursing home shuffle hastily around the room, alternately observing how residents respond to the robots and keeping the machines from getting damaged in falls. They swap out empty batteries and cycle robots in and out to keep residents as engaged as possible.

The relative immobility of the residents and flurry of activity around them create a kind of theater-in-the-round, with residents as critical audience, robots as actors, and team members as stage managers (see figure 3.2). The theater generates excitement through the spectacle of whirring and whizzing machines. The audience is encouraged to observe, comment, and interact. Residents point at, laugh at, and talk about the robots, much as they try to feel them—touching, touch, pushing, pulling, holding, and petting. Conversation is expected to break out between residents and members of the team, in an imagined way between residents and robots, and, ideally, among residents themselves. Even when robots failed, they succeeded. If they fell over or off the table, they became objects of laughter, robot actors doing robot slapstick.

As Okada-san remarked after one session concluded, being in nursing care places one in a near-constant state of dependence on others. This, he suggested, can be hard on a person's sense of dignity, especially when one is

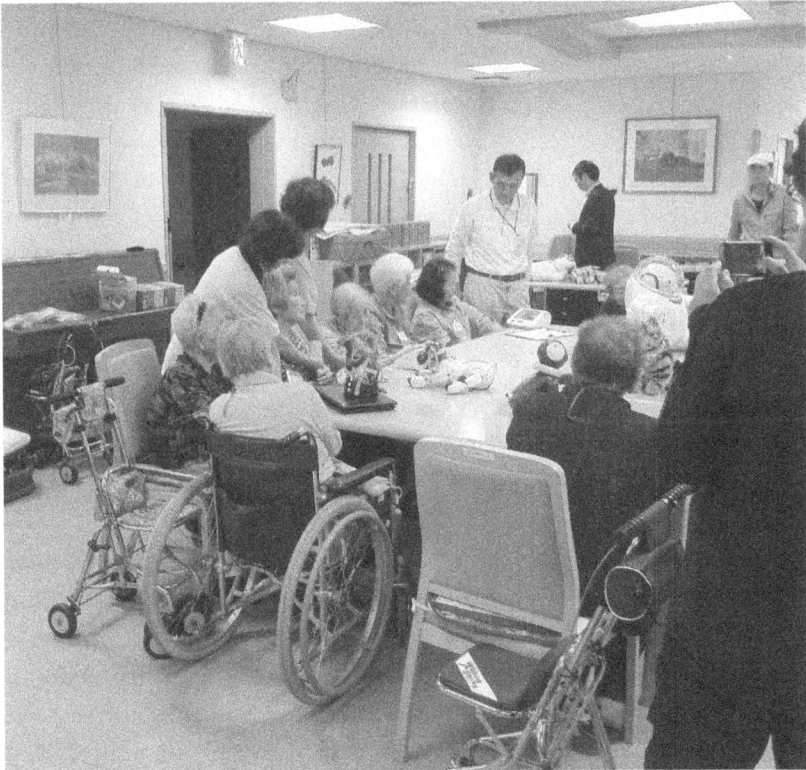

FIGURE 3.2 The Theater of Care.   Members of the Robot Therapy Group and their students facilitate a therapy session with residents at the Leisure Times nursing home. Photo by author.

still conscious of declining cognitive ability. Interacting with an animaloid robot—an object that seems clearly inferior to you—can make you feel superior, more like an adult in control. Indeed, Okada-san stressed that the animal form of the robot is key. "When it looks human," he tells me, "residents tend to stiffen up, thinking that they now have to deal with a person. The etiquette of the human world *(ningen kankei)* applies again. You can't relax and have fun. You must try to behave in line with ordinary rules of propriety."

Animaloid robots here function similarly but not exactly to animals in animal therapy. In animal therapy, of course, it is *animals*, not robots, that are the central focus of activity. And animals attract interest *not* because they perform as something other than an animal; a dog attracts attention *because* it's a dog being a dog. In much the same way, the robots on the table/stage play themselves. Yet, in contrast to animals, the behavior of robots can be much more easily controlled. This can happen in real time, as in the case of the students directly manipulating the AIBO. It can also be programmed in advance. Either way, robots require the work of humans to perform much as humans need robots to create a spectacle beyond what humans can achieve alone. People are just too familiar; robots are not yet that nimble.

The aim of this structured and unstructured activity, members told me, is to create a shared basis for "communication" *(komyunikēshon)*. Despite living together, residents of nursing homes rarely have much in common. They seldom share ties of family, community, occupation, or avocation. They come to the facility for reasons of declining health or decreasing functional independence, not social affinity. Variation in health status means that even if a resident shares an interest with another resident, they may not recognize enough in common to engage in conversation. Living in a group without feeling a sense of community can lead to frustration and hasten the progression of neurodegenerative disease.

An issue stemming from forced collectivity implies a collective solution, and the group makes sure that residents encounter robots together. (Even the individualized attention directed toward the woman I described above occurred at a table she shared with other residents.) At the center of a theatrical round, robots become both objects of enchantment and conversation pieces for people who lack common interests. Importantly, given the varying linguistic competence of residents with dementia, the content of the conversations that emerge is seen as less important than the very *act* of conversing in itself. The Robot Therapy Group privileges this "phatic function" of linguistic exchange—its capacity to affirm social ties without necessarily conferring meaning.[8] Residents might not understand what other residents say. Even if they do, the exchange might quickly be forgotten. Of greater importance is the moment of connection that it affords. These moments are believed to have therapeutic value insofar as they provide relief from feelings of dislocation and social isolation.

In sessions of robot therapy, then, the machines provide infrastructure for engagement. As an assemblage of material objects, the multitude of robots mediates interactions happening around them. By coming between, the robots draw residents together both with each other and with staff as well as therapists. But the mediation is not just physical. Those devices with open operating systems *digitally* mediate human–human interaction while masking the act of mediation itself. Remote-controlled AIBO robots move *as if* they are acting autonomously. Ultimately, the therapeutic effect of sessions depends surprisingly little on the capacity of any particular robot to sense or respond, of any particular feeling machine to feel. Instead, in providing a technological infrastructure for engagement, therapy robots become something other than (semi-)autonomous machines; they become *platforms* for socialization as care.

Robot Therapy as Experiment

At the end of the session, residents were wheeled out of the room one by one. Tables and chairs were returned to their proper spots. Papers, clipboards, worksheets, video cameras, and laptops were gathered up. Robots were carried downstairs and packed into boxes for shipping back to Prof. Matsuda's office. The team would head downstairs as well, and settle in around the same conference table where they had prepared for the session. Okada-san and a nurse soon arrived with coffee and snacks and new worksheets to distribute. Packing away of computers, routers, robots, and routers to make room for pen and paper had obvious practical importance. But it signaled as well a change in modality—from digital to analog—in the *hanseikai,* or post-activity meeting and discussion.

The worksheet Okada-san circulated was structured like a spreadsheet. The names of residents who had participated in the day's session day ran down a vertical column on the left. Each column to the right corresponded to a particular demographic characteristic (i.e., age, gender) or level of LTCI support.[9] There were additional cells to record which robots an individual interacted with and what kind of emotional expression they displayed. But the primary focus of the worksheet, and of the discussion at the *hanseikai*, was to determine and record the "comprehensive evaluation" score *(sōgō-hyōka)* on a scale from one to five. This effectively converted the assemblage of humans and machines we had just seen in the session into a collection of individualized data selves (Lupton 2019) constructed out of demographic details and clinical indices.

The worksheet, then, operated as more than a mere record of information. It was a vital technological link in transforming a therapeutic session into an experiment that generates data. It served as an "inscription device," to use the terminology of the science studies scholars Bruno Latour and Steve Woolgar. Whereas Latour and Woolgar use this term to describe how scientific instruments transform "pieces of matter into written documents" (1986, 51), the worksheet transforms *immaterial* affects and behavior into numerical inscriptions. Like the laboratories of natural scientists, once an inscription is generated, "all the intermediary steps which made its production possible are forgotten" (Latour and Woolgar 1986, 61). A critical intermediary step is the *hanseikai* itself. Comprehensive evaluation scores are not arrived at merely by asking a session participant how they feel or by checking measurements on a scientific instrument. Determining the nature and intensity of affective expression is a product of observation, analysis, and discussion. Such are the attendant challenges of interpreting the feelings of people whose self-reports are near impossible to ascertain or so inconsistent as to be unreliable. I always came away impressed by how insightful these discussions were, and by how flexibly members of the group shifted between structuring sessions, facilitating interaction, and reflecting on their results. Still, it was hard not to see as well that *hanseikai* reduced the messiness of observable behavior to the kind of numerical data preferred by engineers.

Hanseikai followed a consistent pattern. Okada-san would read an individual participant's name from the worksheet and the group would discuss their reactions. Discussion would continue until the group arrived at a consensus about where to rank the participant's comprehensive evaluation. The group relied on observable engagement and expressive behaviors. The ability to respond to what was happening in the session—in nearly any form—were of central interest, as the cases of participants Y–san and I–san demonstrate.

Okada: Okay, Y–san (Female, 72, LTCI support level 4, Mobility index B2, Dementia rank 3b). She responds well to just about everything!

Matsuda: Right, up for anything . . .

O: I could tell how excited she was when she heard that today was a robot therapy day. Still, today it seemed like she wanted to help out with cooking but she ended up coming back. Robots won out over the appeal of cooking, I guess!

M: It seemed like she got more engaged the longer the session went on . . .

O: It felt good to see her enjoying herself so much.

M: Okay, Y–san . . . a 4, maybe. Shall we say 5?

O: 4, 4 . . . not quite 5 yet, right? (laughs)

O: Okay, then we have I–san (Female, 94 years old, LTCI level 3, Mobility index A1, Dementia rank 3a). She's normally pretty quiet, reserved. Shall we say a 3?

Nurse: Actually, she really seemed to be enjoying things. She was giggling quite a bit.

O: She was giggling? Emotional expression was good then. Shall we say a 5?

M: Yeah, I was thinking it should be a bit, um, higher . . .

O: Her expression was good. She was laughing a bit. 5 it is.

Even when participants did try to articulate themselves verbally, the content of these utterances was less important than the fact that they indicated proof of recognition and responsiveness.

O: All right, third is H–san (Female, 85 years old, LTCI level 4, Mobility index A2, Dementia rank 3a). She was on the corner of the first table. She really responded well.

Kitayama (female undergraduate student): Yes, at first, she was really captivated by Miyoko [the female-gendered name of one of the AIBO robots]. She was calling her by her name "Miyoko-chan . . ." and asking a lot of questions about the robot.

O: Yes, she asks a lot of questions, even when she's not at robot therapy.

Sato: Yeah, it seemed clear to me that she was interested. She even asked questions to the student assistants. Lots of conversations. At the same time, she seemed a bit flustered when there wasn't someone nearby to answer questions.

O: Um, she was responsive the whole time, right?

S: Yes, she was especially interested in Miyoko.

O: So, maybe a 4?

S: Yes.

If sessions of robot therapy are directed specifically at the treatment of dementia symptoms, the post-activity *hanseikai* make clear that they are also about a broader research agenda and legitimation effort of the Robot Therapy Group. Through *hanseikai* and the inscriptions they generate, the theater of care is retroactively transformed into a laboratory of care technique. Therapy sessions in which robots are employed as platforms for social interaction become platforms for research projects—projects meant, recursively, to evaluate the utility of robot therapy itself. These feedback effects of robot therapy sessions circulate far beyond sites of care. While the embodied selves of nursing home residents remain confined, their data selves, inscribed on paper and loaded onto laptops for processing, travel with the group outside of the walls of Leisure Times. Indeed, a few months after the session recounted above, I would watch these inscriptions reappear as figures in the final presentations of students supervised by members of the Robot Therapy Group. Later, I would read them in the pages of articles published by senior members of the group. Sessions of robot therapy facilitate the transformation of therapist-teachers into researchers and students into graduates, much as they turn robotic pets into care technology and the transient sociality of older adults with dementia into experimental data.

Second Lives of Men and Machines

Robot therapy sessions also give the second lives of retirees-turned-educators renewed value through the production, not just the transmission, of knowledge. The gendered dimensions of this are hard to miss. Care of older adults has historically been the preserve of women in Japan and, for much of this time, sites of eldercare have remained spatially distinct from sites of commerce and industry.[10] These spatial distinctions are overlaid with symbolic weight. As the science studies scholar Maria Puig de la Bellacasa writes, "The work of . . . the maintenance of life has traditional been considered marginal to value-creating work" (Puig de la Bellacasa 2015, 708). The femininized work of maintaining life unfolds in a quotidian way not according to the rigid clock time of workdays or the linear timelines of profit maximization.

The elongated meantime of care work expands and contracts organically in response to the rhythms and demands of biological life. Puig de la Bellacasa reminds us, "Care time suspends the future and distends the present, thickening it with a myriad of demanding attachments" (Puig de la Bellacasa 2015, 707). The distended present of everyday care work contrasts sharply with the iterative futurism of the Robot Therapy Group. I do not mean to diminish the commitment of the group to the care of dementia. But their continual tinkering with techniques and machines, the integration of their activities into supervised student projects, and their own aspirations as researchers seem at odds with any suspension of the future.

If the gendered dimensions of their activities differ from the traditional work of care, so, too, does the composition of its membership. I never saw a woman colleague involved in the planning or execution of any robot therapy session. In fact, the only women I observed participating were the students of professors in the group. The uniformly male cast of robot therapists could not differ more from the institutionalized subjects of their care, who are overwhelmingly female. When asked about the obvious gender imbalance, members would say that it was really no surprise given the male dominance of engineering professions in Japan (especially robotics engineers). Additionally, and perhaps more revealingly, they would lament that few women researchers, or women care workers, had demonstrated much interest in their activities.

I have already noted that sessions are led by men who concluded successful careers as salaried workers in some of Japan's largest business conglomerates. The chronology of their careers aligns with the country's ascendance as a global economic power. Their technical expertise clusters around one of the technologies (robots) closely identified with the muscularity of Japan's industrial capitalism in the twentieth century, their careers forged by harnessing those machines to productive ends. Now, perhaps ironically, they find themselves enrolled in the care of an older, and overwhelmingly female, surfeit of bodies—a population both created by and dependent on the shared affluence their labor helped to produce.

In striving to make their care work productive, the leaders of the Robot Therapy Group resist the gendered loss of status that accompanies the transition from corporate work to care work. They elide the transition by applying a surplus of skills honed in the former toward the care of surplus life in the latter. Their commitment to using machines might then be understood sympathetically, rather than dismissed as the intrusion of "cold" technology into "warm" relations of human caregiving (an opposition coded with gendered assumptions; see Aulino 2016). Generating opportunities for connection and enhancing psychological well-being are their primary objectives. Doing so with mediating machines is an effort to care but in a distinctly masculine mode. Whether the wider use of care robotics will draw more men into the profession remains to be seen. For the older leaders of the group, however, robot therapy is more than just an iterative engagement of older adults and robotics technology. It is a masculinized platform through which aging engineers can construct a life 2.0 in a post-retirement landscape of care.

Robot Therapy 2.0

On subsequent short visits to Japan in 2012, 2014, and 2015, I observed multiple additional sessions of robot therapy. The changes to them were mostly incremental—students conducted new experiments; new robots were introduced; elements of the session were subtly adjusted. On a visit in fall 2017, however, I noticed that the structure of robot therapy sessions had changed significantly. In this robot therapy 2.0, the platformization of robots that I had observed previously had intensified. Rather than being marginalized to student experimentation, the robot-as-platform had become the focus of the activity.

Change was apparent as soon as I arrived at Leisure Times. Okada-san ushered us into the conference room where the group usually prepares. I did not see boxes of robots that had been sent in advance. Instead, as we entered, I spotted a rack of three wire shelves that were filled with robots that the group now used routinely. Among the familiar AIBO, Paro, and NeCoRo robots, there was a new arrival, a robot called Yumenoko Neruru. This robot is an entertainment robot—basically a talking doll—manufactured by a company called Takara Tomy A.R.T.S. It is a feeling machine *par excellence*: like Paro, it activates when it is touched. When its hands are squeezed, it recites set phrases and plays songs. In addition to the new robots, two postdoctoral engineers had joined the team. The additional labor support enabled the group to increase the frequency of its visits to Leisure Times to as often as once a week.

The effect of these human and nonhuman additions became clear when I saw how they had modified the robot therapy sessions from just a few years prior. As we chatted, the postdocs checked that batteries in each of the baby

doll robots were full. They test-squeezed the robots' hands, triggering programmed phrases and songs. One played with hair on one of the dolls, spik-
ing it up comically in the fashion of an anime character. Another fit a harness
on the team's newest AIBO and a name tag on it that read "lucky" *(rakki)* in
Japanese *katakana* script.

We moved upstairs together and entered the usual activity space. The
group began setting up two large tables about ten feet apart, leaving a much
larger space in the center of the room than I had seen previously. They placed
a wooden pallet in this space and began assembling what looked to be a
miniature arena out of interlocking rubber flooring. The tiled arena would
feature prominently in the latter half of the session. The group placed its
collection of baby doll robots on another table pushed against a wall. Next
to it, they stacked about a dozen small, square crates. They also set up two
video cameras on opposite sides of the room and launched a temporary WiFi
network. Gone were the laptops that had previously featured so centrally.
The group's technology had "advanced" to include an iPad that performed
many of the control functions of older laptops but in a portable and much less
conspicuous form.

Prof. Matsuda explained that the group's approach to these activity sessions had evolved as well. Instead of just having the residents sit around the
table with various robots lying in front of them and interacting with them
as they might like, the group structured the activity in three parts. Matsuda
explained that the new approach let the residents "get used to" *(narete kuru)*
the robots for about twenty minutes before they played a game and exercised
together. He explained that the inclusion of exercise was inspired by new research he had read on the positive effect that physical activity could have on
the psychological well-being of people with dementia.

Soon residents began to file in and were positioned around the tables.
Once they found a place, one of the team would put a Yumenoko Neruru
doll in front of them. The member would briefly explain how to operate the
device. Soon after, most of the residents began to interact very quickly, listening intently to the phrases coming out of the speaker and smiling back at the
(perpetually) smiling robot. Nearly all thirteen residents who participated
had a doll in front of them. Those who did not were presented with a Paro
robot or with one of the AIBO.

A few minutes later, Prof. Matsuda and his younger assistant, Dr. Inoguchi, announced the start of another activity. I quickly learned the purpose

of the square crates I had seen stacked next to the equipment table. The group filled half of them with around twenty orange-colored ping-pong balls and half with white ping-pong balls. They gathered the residents around the makeshift arena. "Lucky" the AIBO robot sat waiting in the center of the arena. Before positioning Lucky there, the team had attached an empty plastic crate atop his back.

The team divided the full crates among the residents, placing them on their laps. Inoguchi announced that the group was now going to play a game called "Tama-ire." He explained that residents were to throw as many of their ping-pong balls into the container on "Lucky-chan's" back as they could, until he blew a whistle to end the activity.[11] At the conclusion of the game, the group would count the number of ping-pong balls in the container. The team with the most balls, either orange or white, would win. Blowing a whistle, Inoguchi signaled the start of the game. Immediately, residents began tossing balls toward the container on the back of Lucky. Inoguchi held an iPad in his hands and watched the action carefully. A set of virtual pushbuttons was visible on its screen. Pushing one of these buttons triggered preprogrammed movements in the AIBO robot, much like the group used laptops in the past. By triggering the robot in this way, Inoguchi could control the flow of the game such that both sides had an equal opportunity to get their balls in the container.

The process was working well when in the middle of the game, Lucky-*chan* advanced too far forward and began to fall off the floor of the arena. Dr. Inoguchi and his colleagues swept in quickly to set Lucky-*chan* upright, and the game continued. Lucky-*chan*'s fall provided a momentary comedic break in the action; robot slapstick never seems to get old. Except for a couple of individuals who seemed to have difficulty following the action, the residents were intensely focused on the game and worked hard to complete their throws into the container. The activity instantly transformed the loose collection of individuals into teams working in tandem, the atmosphere charged with competitive intensity. Members of the group did help residents when they ran into difficulty, but they tended to intervene less than in previous sessions I observed. This was a time for the residents to work together intentionally toward a specific goal, albeit within the structure of an organized activity.

The game finished with a lopsided result: the team with the orange ping-pong balls routed the team with the white ones. Even so, Dr. Inoguchi dramatically pulled each ball out of the basket one at a time. He made a show of counting slowly, demonstrably holding each ball up for the residents to see like he had just found a precious gem—"Hitotsu, futatsu, mitsu . . ." (One, Two, Three . . .). Those residents who could counted along with him. Counting out loud together, the group operated as a collective once again, reenacting one of the classic activities of primary school. No prizes were awarded, nor was there any meaningful recognition of the team that had won, save for a brief mention of the winning side.

Soon after the game had concluded, Dr. Inoguchi declared that the group would now do robot-led "radio exercises" *(rajio taisō)*. Radio exercises are a set of calisthenics that are broadcast every morning on radio in Japan. The routine is always the same; the idea is to encourage daily exercise by everyone. Residents were surely familiar with these exercises since childhood. Three AIBO robots had been programmed to move along with the tune that accompanies radio exercises. From their seats, residents mimed the movements of the robot to the best of their ability, many of them struggling to raise their arms and rotate their bodies like the robot dogs. The exercises lightened the mood and provided a break from the intense concentration required by the *tama-ire* game, but they still kept the group of residents active and engaged.

Of course, one of the regular nursing staff could have guided the residents instead of the robots. (When they could, staff did join in.) But then, it would have seemed like just another activity. The novelty of having the robot do these movements gave this part of the session meaning beyond the kinds of everyday care provided by the human staff members. Residents moved in synchrony with the robot according to a deeply familiar cultural script, reenacting movements learned long ago. Recreation became *re*-creation. Unlike the "theater-in-the-round" I had seen previously, residents did not pause to laugh at or comment about the robots. They followed feeling machines when the robots were reduced to their most robotic, carrying out programmed instructions without reacting to the people around them.

Once radio exercises concluded, the team repeated the *tama-ire* game and ended with robot-led radio exercises once more. This was enough activity for the day. Staff gradually wheeled those who looked tired out of the room and back to their usual spot in the cafeteria. Prof. Matsuda positioned another AIBO robot on a table at the center of the room. The robot played the institution's theme song and danced along to its rhythms. A couple of women stayed after, chatting with members of the team. "How was it?" one of the team asked her. "Oh, I am so happy *(ureshii)*," she answered. "I worked up a good sweat *(ase bisshori)*." She watched the robot move along to the beat of the theme song. "Good! Good! *(jōzu jōzu)*," she said in admiration. She looked over at another woman who was holding one of the Yumenoko Neruru dolls. "It looks real, doesn't it?" she asked. The woman with the doll smiled but otherwise didn't signal agreement. Instead, she seemed captivated by the robot she was holding. "Is this a girl? It looks like a girl," she asked aloud to no one in particular. By this time, members of the Robot Therapy Group had started packing up and were distracted by their work. The woman straightened out the clothes on the robot, and gently lifted its dress up to take a quick peek. Her curiosity apparently satisfied, she quickly laid the dress back down, brushing her hand over it a couple of times, as if to straighten out any wrinkles and apologize for any transgression. She handed the doll to a member of the group standing nearby, who then wheeled her and the other women out of the room. They said a final goodbye to Lucky-*chan*. Inoguchi called after them, giving Lucky-*chan* a voice when the robot could not produce its own: "Come play with me again!"

Prof. Matsuda told me later he believed the new sequencing of the therapy session (i.e., dolls, *tama-ire* game, radio exercises) was one of the most significant revisions to robot therapy since its inception. It more effectively eased a diverse group of residents into interaction than the looser structure of sessions in the past. Yet, even though the structure of the session may have changed, its aim remained the same. The group worked to orchestrate an encounter that elicited affects of enchantment and excitement while also generating moments of solidarity and social interaction, all in an effort to reduce the stress of living in relative social isolation. This "robot therapy 2.0" builds on and intensifies the use of robots with open operating systems, like AIBO, as platforms for social engagement that I observed in past sessions. In the makeshift arena, Lucky-*chan* became both a material platform—supporting an empty crate—and an immaterial one that helped trigger affective responses and channel social engagement.

Worksheets and collective quantification of emotion in post-activity *hanseikai* were also conserved but in streamlined form. Okada-san and a nurse arrived in the conference room, circulated worksheets, read through the names, and facilitated a discussion about the reactions of the residents. But this time the group only recorded whether a person reacted positively or not, a binary choice devoid of the numerical gradations of the past. Worksheets still included scores from past sessions, an important element in sustaining the group's ethos of continuous experimentation. The list of numbers symbolized as well that this day was one of many in the past and in the future to come, a series without predefined end.

Worksheets completed, the team discussed what had gone well and what still needed work. They debated how better to arrange the space to prevent Lucky-*chan* from falling over, how to keep balls from flying out of the arena, how to ensure equity of outcomes between the teams. They spent even more time trying to figure out how best to capture the effect that interacting with robots had on residents. Someone suggested choosing one or two residents to regularly follow and record during the activity. This solution generated some interest, but it also introduced a potential problem: what would be the best position for a camera meant to capture a resident's expression without interfering in their participation? The team could not know whether a resident would look directly at the camera or for long enough. And even if they did capture these expressions accurately, their interpretations of them would remain insufficient, frustratingly subjective. Perhaps, Prof. Matsuda suggested, they could employ new AI to analyze the facial expressions using machine learning. He added, trying to be helpful, that he knew a start-up that had created just this kind of software application. In fact, at another nursing home, the group had already tried out a similar computerized speech recognition system. Residents recited a series of phrases before and after robot therapy, and then the system algorithmically evaluated whether there were any effects on verbal fluency. Prof. Matsuda's younger colleagues paused to consider the option, their expressions signaling neither assent nor outright dismissal.

The exchange, mundane as it was, evoked the past and hinted at the future. Prof. Matsuda began a career in robotics, awed by technology's ability to move people beyond natural limits but wary of its equally capacious potential to fail and cause harm. His efforts in robot therapy attempted to overcome limitations of both the human and the technological in the service of caring for the end of life. Might technology once again help the team overcome a hurdle that remained; that is, accounting for the effect of robot therapy on the feelings of others? Ultimately, the issue was tabled. Perhaps the group would try it; perhaps they would try something else. For a professor nearing the conclusion of his own second life, the question would be left for the young men sitting across from him. This irresolution signaled not failure or disagreement but a moment for yet another iteration of robot therapy to begin, again.

———

Unresolved, indeed. Gotō-san, one of the oldest members of the team, sat next to me on a train back to Tokyo after one session of robot therapy. Out of nowhere, he turned to me and said, "You know, I got tenure at the age of eighty-one because I am a good singer." At first, I thought he was joking, but it turned out that he sings opera as a hobby and performs for students at his school's annual opening ceremony. When officials from the Ministry of Education, Sports, Culture, Science and Technology recently visited the school, they asked his supervisors why they employ an eighty-one-year-old tenured professor. "He sings," they said. "It's interesting." He winked at me, "I never thought singing would come in so handy."

The train sped down the tracks, jostling mildly from side to side. Gotō-san looked my way again again. "So, recently we had a professor from another university visit a research group at my school to give a presentation about the meaning of happiness *(shiawase)*. She talked about how *ureshii, tanoshii,* and *shiawase* [related words for "happy" in Japanese] are in fact different. You see, *ureshii* or *tanoshii* is something that you feel at a moment in time, like 'happy,' but *shiawase* is a state of mind, more like 'happiness.' She told us that she had been doing additional research into whether people with dementia experience happiness *(shiawase)*."

"Do you want to know her answer," he asked.

"Sure. What was it?"

"*Wakaranai*," she said. "Nobody knows."

FOUR

Embracing Paro

In Denmark, happiness is a point of national pride. Danes are quick to tell you that they are among the happiest people the world, and this is not just idle boasting: Denmark routinely places toward the top on global surveys of life satisfaction like the UN-supported World Happiness Report.[1]

When you ask why, it's rare to hear reference to national character, good humor, or pleasant weather. Instead, Danes tend to attribute overall well-being to provisions of their welfare state: taxpayer-supported cradle-to-grave healthcare, free public education through graduate school, five weeks annual paid vacation, lengthy parental leave, subsidized daycare and eldercare, among other benefits. The answer is a revealing glimpse into collective consciousness. It suggests that happiness is not a feeling that individuals generate for themselves regardless of circumstances external to them. People feel happy when they are cared for by the community in which they live. Good care makes people happy; if people are happy, it means that they are receiving good care.

Of course, a good welfare state depends on a sufficient tax base to support it. While Denmark's proportion of older adults is not nearly as high as it is in Japan, low fertility rates have generated similar anxiety about the pressure of population aging on the future of the welfare state. This has led to politically fraught calls for neoliberal reform as well as nativist hostility toward immigrants from the Global South, whom some believe dilute the capacity of the state to care for its citizens. Less controversially, it has intensified interest in what the Danes call "welfare technologies" *(velfærdsteknologi)*. Like *fukushi-kiki* in Japan, welfare technologies are defined performatively: they are digital technologies used in the delivery of social welfare services. The belief is that effective welfare technology could help the state to do more with less, decreasing the cost of welfare without sacrificing quality (Dahler 2018). Aggressive investment in welfare technology also signals that the state is taking action in the present to address what seems like an unavoidable crisis of the future.

In Denmark, then, a robot that helps older adults feel happy would likely be attractive to both government and the public at large. Indeed, Paro the robot seal from Japan is used throughout Denmark in the care of older adults with dementia. This chapter explores, first, how Paro has been incorporated into Danish dementia care and, second, how Danish dementia care has guided the technological development of Paro. I argue that the appropriation of Paro by care professionals in Denmark began the iterative process by which Paro was transformed from a robot meant to be kept as a pet to one with a primarily therapeutic application. It is no exaggeration to say that the identification of Paro with dementia care originates in Denmark, not Japan. This close engagement continues as of this writing, if less intensely than at the start.

In Denmark, as in Japan, Paro mediates interactions between care workers and residents with dementia. However, those interactions take place more often in one-on-one settings than in groups, and Danish dementia care focuses much more explicitly on the enhancement of "quality of life" *(livskvalitet)*. Enhancing quality of life (QoL) is typically understood in an individual sense; that is, the raising of one resident's QoL through a successful interaction with Paro. Yet, for reasons I will discuss in more detail, maintaining individualized QoL in nursing homes assumes added significance in the specific cultural context of Danish nursing care, where taking coercive action to modify the behavior of a resident with dementia is tightly circumscribed. Paro, the fuzzy seal robot, becomes part of a distributed infrastructure of nursing care that works to maintain order within nursing homes by minimizing the expression of negative affect. In Denmark, encounters of Paro and patients help keep older adults happy and nursing homes running smoothly.

Successful or unsuccessful encounters, furthermore, drive the iterative development of the robot itself.

Paro for Dementia Care

"In Denmark, we have more Paro per capita than anywhere else in the world, even Japan!" Olivia, the leader of the one-day certification workshop on caring with Paro that I attended in the summer of 2012, announced to a group of mostly women care workers seated in a semicircle in front of her. The workshop was being held in Odense, a city in western Denmark about a hundred miles from Copenhagen, at the headquarters of the Danish Technological Institute (DTI). DTI is a nonprofit consultancy firm that helps identify and promote emerging technologies for target markets in Denmark and Europe. At the time, DTI was the central distribution hub for Paro throughout Europe. Most attendees that day had been sent by care facilities in Denmark that wished to purchase Paro, but there were some participants from nearby Sweden as well. The certification workshop, which cost 500 euros, was effectively mandatory since DTI only sold Paro to care facilities with at least two licensed staff members. It was also the first of its kind, and without any Japanese model. Olivia pioneered the certificate workshop after helping run a pilot program that introduced Paro into nursing homes around Copenhagen. The success of that pilot program—the "Paro Project"—encouraged the Danish government to purchase over one hundred Paro, leading to the outsized presence of the Japanese robot in Danish nursing homes and dementia-care centers.

Olivia is trained as a physical therapist and also has a degree in education. She already had over thirty years of experience working among older adults with dementia when I met her at the workshop. In an interview later in 2017, she told me that she finds working with older adults to be more interesting than working with young people. "[Older adults] typically have more than one specific problem. It's always a combination of things. To me, it's very challenging to find out what to focus on, what kind of treatment should the individual have. When you're old, it's always a combination of problems. Physical, cognitive, this and that . . . I don't see the body as some surface, I see the body as deeply connected to the mind."

Olivia's expertise in dementia care eventually led to membership in the

Behavioral and Psychological Symptoms of Dementia task force for the city of Copenhagen. The task force visited institutions or homes where care workers were facing challenges in dementia care, typically individuals who were aggressive or noncompliant in one form or another. Around 2004, the city of Copenhagen launched the "Be Safe Project" *(Vær Tryg-projektet)*, which aimed to test the effectiveness of dozens of technologies to assist with the care of such individuals. While working on that project, Olivia saw a newspaper article on the Paro robot and its inventor, Takanori Shibata, who had just visited Denmark to present his device at a product expo for healthcare aids. Olivia immediately recognized the potential of the Paro robot for dementia care. She contacted Dr. Shibata and asked if she could get some Paro to try in therapy.

> He told me, "Well, it's a Japanese technology for people who can't take care of their pet dogs anymore. They buy it for their own amusement." But I told him, "Oh, I think Paro might be a therapeutic tool, and I'd like to buy some." He told me that he would have to check, "We are very interested in selling Paro but it's not quite ready for export yet." You know, when we got the first Paros, they had the wrong adapters and we couldn't use them. I had to take them to an electrician to have them converted for use with Danish electrical outlets. Eventually, when we ordered more, Takanori [Shibata] heard about this issue and changed the adapters for us! (laughs)

It was not just the adapters that needed adjustment. Paro had a new purpose.

Paro is now used so frequently in dementia care that it is hard to imagine a time when this was not its primary purpose. At least how it appeared in media reports to Olivia, Paro was still mainly a substitute pet, like the robot cat (NeCoRo), on which Dr. Shibata worked during his time at the Omron corporation, and Sony's AIBO robot before it. Even then, the idea of using animaloid robots in care was not entirely new. The Robot Therapy Group in Japan regularly used AIBO and NeCoRo in nursing homes before Olivia first read about Paro (see chapter 3). Shibata and colleagues had already examined the effect of interacting with Paro on older adults, though not specifically for the treatment of dementia (Wada et al. 2002a, 2002b). These studies led to Paro being designated the "World's Most Therapeutic Robot" by Guinness World Records in 2002.[2] Still, Olivia suggested that the therapeutic application of Paro in dementia care derived from its Danish experience.

S: When you met Dr. Shibata, he said that Paro was meant for entertainment, not just for older adults with dementia?

O: Right. What happened was that Shibata got very interested in our
project. It seemed to me that the therapeutic way of using Paro was
new to him . . . But the moment he got the idea, you know, he went
around to different nursing homes in Denmark and other countries . . .
and Paro is now more a therapeutic tool than, say, someone's pet dog.

Danish media quickly learned of Paro's integration into the Be Safe Project. Journalists and television crews soon accompanied Olivia's team as they
trialed Paro and other technologies for care. Their reports helped popular-
ize Paro as Denmark's "first robot for eldercare." The association between
Paro and Denmark would soon become global. Coincidentally, as Olivia was
testing Paro in Denmark, the Danish director Phie Ambo was filming a documentary in Japan on roboticist Ishiguro Hiroshi's experiments with hyper-
realistic androids. The process of making the documentary brought Ambo
into contact with Dr. Shibata, who introduced her to Paro and to a couple
in Japan who had purchased one as a pet. He also told her about Paro's role
in the Be Safe Project. When she returned home, she began following that
project as well. Subtitled in English and distributed internationally, Ambo's
documentary *Mechanical Love* (Ambo 2007) includes segments on the couple
who adopted Paro in Japan as well as Olivia's work with Paro in a Copenhagen nursing home. Ambo's work further cemented the association of Paro
with dementia care in Demark.

Following the successful conclusion of the Be Safe Project in 2008, national and local governments directed public funds to the purchase of more
Paro. No other country, not even Paro's home country of Japan, had pursued
the robot so enthusiastically. Japanese manufacturers of Paro contracted with
DTI to coordinate the sale and distribution of Paro in Europe and to collect
data on its implementation. DTI consultants relied so often on Olivia's expertise in introducing nursing-home staff to the capabilities of Paro that they
eventually hired her on fulltime as a consultant on a new "Paro Project."
(This project ran from 2008 through 2012, when I first met Olivia, until 2014).
Olivia drew on her experience with Paro and her training as an educator to
design a mandatory Paro certification course. In addition to DTI's efforts
and prior to its distribution throughout the country, Denmark's Council on
Ethics approved Paro for use in dementia care.[3] The council concluded that

Paro would not cause harm if used correctly, but cautioned that Paro should not substitute for human contact or caregiving. They made no determination on the robot's efficacy.

Paro's path into Danish care is notable for the way in which it deviates from deterministic narratives of technological adoption. Paro was not an existing tool for dementia care that happened to be taken up in Denmark. Olivia saw new potential in the robot. She helped devise new ways of using it in the delivery of dementia care. The process transformed Paro into something it had not yet been. Paro's identity as a technology for dementia care now became entangled with the people and practices of the Danish welfare state.

What was it that initially attracted Olivia to Paro? Partly, it was its appearance. Back in the certification workshop, Olivia compares the robot Paro with video of an actual baby harp seal filmed by Dr. Shibata in Canada. She points out the significant changes. Gone are the sharp teeth in the actual seal, which might be threatening. Large eyes, much larger than an actual baby seal, are key to eliciting the nonverbal communication that is vital to dementia care. Paro makes squeals sampled from actual recordings of baby harp seals, minus the aggressive sounds they can make. Paro also cannot move through physical space on its own. Its head, body, and paws do move, but much more slowly and gently than an actual seal. Its fur is soft and it does not respond aggressively when touched. These modifications combine to make Paro much less threatening than a wild animal.[4] "Whether he intended to or not, Takanori [Shibata] designed a robot with a user interface that is brilliant. It is so cute, with a round face, big eyes, and a small mouth without the sharp teeth," Olivia tells me later.

Also vital is the functional emphasis Paro places on interaction. "Paro can't do anything on its own," Olivia stresses. Unlike AIBO, it cannot be directed to perform in any specific way by a care professional. Touch and the response to touch are key to its functionality and efficacy. Its size and furry exterior encourage an intimate embrace. Olivia continues, "It's the feeling of touching something, being next to something. [Gesturing to her lap and lower abdomen] Paro lies right here where you have a special connection. It's where the pregnant woman has a child, where the woman who has just borne a child sits with it. Touching this area has a strong connection with your feelings, with your memories. When two people are in love, they connect here. It's a special zone . . . This is one of the biggest features of Paro, if not the biggest." Among care workers I met, there was broad agreement that Paro's capacity to elicit and respond to tactile interaction set it apart from other nonresponsive objects, like dolls, that are commonly used in dementia care. Paro can sit with you. It can lie close to your body. It can respond to your touch. Paro is a machine that feels. It is made to be felt and it makes you feel.

Caring for Quality of Life

As a feeling machine, Paro assists care workers in delivering good dementia care. Paro helps bring a sense of calm to older adults with dementia. This in turn helps accomplish an equally important objective of Danish dementia care: the enhancement of quality of life. Care workers often treated these two dimensions of subjective experience—positive affect and QoL—as equivalent.

The emphasis on QoL among the elderly derives from the commitment of dementia professionals in Denmark to what is often called "person-centered care" (Kontos 2005). Care workers I met drew inspiration from work of the English psychologist Thomas Kitwood. In the 1980s and 1990s, Kitwood's published work challenged dominant understandings of dementia as a malady that results solely from neurological degeneration. The expression of symptoms and the progression of disease, Kitwood argued, depends importantly on the social context in which the person with dementia finds himself. Social milieu that are not responsive to the needs and desires of persons with dementia can exacerbate the expression of antisocial behaviors or even hasten the tendency to self-harm. Conversely, social contexts that try to validate the needs and wants of those with dementia can reduce such tendencies. The title of Kitwood's book *Dementia Reconsidered: The Person Comes First* (1997) expresses in summary form the emphasis on personhood in his work. In Kitwoodian terms, there are no "dementia sufferers" or "demented elderly" (even though these terms sometimes appear in his own writing), rather there are "*persons* with dementia." Personhood is not lost; people are not their diagnosis.[5]

The implications for care practice are clear. If a person with dementia is exhibiting what have come to be called behavioral and psychological symptoms of dementia—the very kinds of things that Olivia and her team worked on prior to her participation in the Be Safe Project—then the care worker ought to adjust aspects of the social environment that are failing to satisfy the person. In Kitwood's view, all people with dementia have an abiding need for love. In addition, he sees five psychological needs as particularly important: the need for comfort, the need for social bonding or attachment, the desire to be included in social life, the need to be occupied in meaningful activity, and the need to maintain a continuous sense of identity (Kitwood 1997, 19–20). "The prime task of dementia care," Kitwood writes, "is to maintain personhood in the face of . . . failing mental powers . . . [and] through the sensitive meeting of this cluster of needs . . . in a way that corresponds to the uniqueness of each individual" (Kitwood 1997, 20)

In Denmark, Kitwood's ideas resonate with the deeply held belief that autonomy must be respected at all stages of the life course. Staff in the institutions that I visited stressed the importance of respecting the right to self-determination for all residents with dementia, regardless of incapacitation. Such respect is reflected in the words used to describe persons under their care. Individuals with dementia were never called "patients," which would have the effect of prioritizing their disease and reinforcing the biomedical orientation of hospital care. Nor were they called "residents," which can connote a kind of transient institutional identity. Instead, when talking with me in English, staff and administrators referred to them as "citizens" (a translation of the Danish *borgere*), affirming their status as persons who need care but who maintain rights granted by the state.[6] Where the social welfare system ensures that "citizens live their lives in and out of state institutions" (Svendsen et al. 2018, 23), the intentional use of citizen residents reminds Danish care workers that the move to institutional care represents a continuation of the responsibility of the welfare state to support its citizenry, not a disruption. It also means that care workers understand older adults with dementia to be capable of making choices and decisions, since making one's own choices and decisions is an essential expression, if not an obligation, of Danish citizenship. Good care, in this sense, entails providing for people not what you perceive them to need but what you understand them to want. And one cannot understand the wants of another, hard as it may be to determine in the case of people with dementia, unless one approaches them as a person in an effort to build a social relationship. The importance of the social environment and the relationship between care workers and people with dementia in Kitwood's approach align with this emphasis on agentive personhood.

While interactions between individuals in nursing homes were founded on respect for self-determination, the means and ends of care were often described as a process of self-realization. In a conversation with three female senior staff at a dementia-care center in Copenhagen, one woman, who was a highly educated dementia-care professional for one of Copenhagen's five administrative districts, contrasted poor care with good care:

> You have to communicate with the person with dementia to find out what works. You need to be creative. You need to be a detective. It's not enough to just "do a job" without being creative. Care workers, some of whom are not well educated, sometimes feel more confident—and think that they're a doing a good job—if they just follow written guidelines mechanically, like "I'm supposed to change the diaper. I'm supposed to put the cream on the skin. I'm supposed to make sure that they're clean and showered and look nice." But for people with dementia that doesn't work. I mean of course you still have to do the toothbrush and stuff, but the ultimate goal is well-being, getting the person to a place of well-being.

Having well-being as a target meant moving beyond merely helping a person function as a biological being by assisting with activities of daily living. It meant more than helping a person just live a greater *quantity* of days; it meant helping them live lives of greater *quality* (Gjødsbøl, Koch, and Svendsen 2017, 117). Ultimately, if done correctly, the dichotomy of quantity and quality breaks down. Helping individuals achieve quality of life, a sense of well-being, helps to slow, but of course never entirely reverse, the progression of an incurable disease.

Putting Paro into Practice

It was in this—facilitating the achievement of quality of life—that care workers saw the therapeutic value of Paro.[7] Touching Paro, holding Paro, cuddling Paro, talking to Paro, talking about Paro, responding to Paro—all manner of interacting with Paro held the potential to increase QoL for citizens. In interviews, the vital importance of QoL appeared so often in the accounts of nursing home staff that I stopped making special note of it. But how exactly did care workers use Paro with citizens in order to raise QoL and how did they assess whether interaction with Paro had indeed raised QoL? Answering these questions, I suggest, begins with recognizing how achieving quality of life *qua* happiness functions doubly in Danish nursing homes, first, as the desired outcome of individually oriented care and, second, as the affective basis on which nursing homes run smoothly.

Care workers noted that they tried to use Paro with people who seem discontented, agitated, or aggressive. On a visit to a nursing home in Køge, a municipality about twenty-five miles southwest of Copenhagen, Anne, the director, invites me to observe how Paro is used by two individuals who have advanced cases of dementia. We stop by Inger's room who, I am told, is not able to do anything on her own. She rarely speaks and usually sits with her fists clenched. When we enter her room, Anne tells me that Inger has just been given a bath. Moments later, Kristina, a female staff member, arrives with a Paro robot. Kristina crouches down and presents Paro to Inger. She places Paro on her lap so that Inger can put her hands on it. Kristina sits next to Inger, close enough that she can touch both Inger and the robot. This kind of one-on-one interaction with Paro as technological mediator was similar to the structure of most interactions that I saw in Denmark. In contrast to Japan, where the Robot Therapy Group uses multiple robots with multiple residents in a common space, care workers in Denmark tended to use Paro alone in more individualized contexts. They would bring Paro to the residents, into their rooms or to them when they were sitting in a public space.

Immediately after receiving Paro, Inger starts hugging Paro tightly and begins to moan. Her interaction with Paro lasts about fifteen minutes, and during this time Inger doesn't talk at all. Anne and Kristina tell me that Inger usually only speaks a few words here and there. Sometimes she will even burst out crying or will start to whine for no apparent reason. However, when they present Paro to her, they tell me that interacting with the robot "gives her comfort" and "calms her down." They bring Paro to her daily, and she tends not to whine if she has had time with Paro. The interaction between Inger (the citizen) and Paro (the robot) is tactile, visual, and aural. It lasts only fifteen minutes because otherwise the stimulation would overwhelm Inger and she would stop responding.

Aside from moaning, Inger doesn't talk to Paro. But Kristina talks with Inger and to Paro throughout the interaction. Kristina rubs Inger's shoulders and strokes her arm, forging tactile connection through her hands just as Inger does with Paro. At one point, while I am looking down writing notes, Anne and Kristina both gasp and tell me to look. Paro had kicked one of its paws and Inger tried to comfort it. This interaction—Inger responding to Paro's movement—was seen as a highlight of the session with Paro and an example of Paro's appeal compared to other kinds of dementia technology. Paro elicited empathy and recognition in Inger. It was a moment of agency, when the cared for turned into the caring for, whether intentional or not. As they conclude the session, Anne and Kristina tell me that Inger is feeling better. She is calmer, they say, even though I cannot tell myself. The nature of this interaction—both in terms of what happens and how it is described—are emblematic of how sessions with Paro proceed: the emphasis on touch and response; on changing emotional expression from agitated to calm; and on Paro as mediator between citizens and professional care workers.

Anne guides me from Inger's room to that of another woman named Kristen. Anne and Kristen's helper Nina give me a rundown of Kristen's behavioral tendencies. They tell me that Kristen rarely smiles and is unable to interact with other people living in the complex because she finds the stimulation overwhelming. When they present Paro to her, they find that she starts to smile and relax, an effect that tends to last for the rest of the day. They bring Paro daily for about thirty minutes, at which point Kristen starts to tire. Once, they tell me, when Nina was on vacation, a replacement care worker did not regularly bring Paro to Kristen and "she started to withdraw into herself." I see Kristen clutch Paro in her lap from the moment she receives it. She holds Paro tightly (she has more facility with her hands than Inger), strokes the robot's back and rubs her chin on Paro's fur. She looks down at Paro as Paro's head turns up toward her. The session is once again entirely nonverbal, but does appear to make Kristen more aware of her surroundings. She notices that Nina is holding a can of Coke and that she doesn't have one. She indicates that she would like a Coke, too. This lightens the mood. Chuckling, Nina fetches her the drink and concludes the session.

The primacy of tactility in these two interactions is heightened by the inability of these two women to speak. But feeling the robot physically and emotionally, being *affected* by it, is vital even for people who retain some linguistic facility. An interaction between Paro and a woman named Ingrid at a nursing home in Copenhagen's Nørrebro district illustrates this, and demonstrates further how Paro assists in the provision of good care.

Like many I visited, Ingrid's nursing home housed individuals with varying levels of dementia. Those with more severe forms of the disease reside on a higher floor that doubles as a special dementia-care center. Once I arrive, a nurse named Jena takes me to Ingrid's room. Jena tells me as we approach that she asked Ingrid's permission in advance for me to observe. As we enter, I see Ingrid dressed in a gray sweater and navy-blue pants smiling back at us and sitting in a chair. A Paro robot lies in a basket on top of a small wheeled cart in the room. Jena has me sit next to Ingrid and asks her if she would like to try the robot. Ingrid assents, and Jena slowly wheels the cart over to Ingrid, who starts talking to Paro as soon as the robot comes into her view. Ingrid's speech is a mix of Danish words and a kind of babytalk, the sort of speech one might hear when a mother talks to an infant and mimics the sounds babies make on their way to acquiring speech. (I indicate these words below in italics.)

> I: Yeah, it is, the little *musse,* yes, yes. On, no, no. Come here little *musse. Musse* wants to play, *laaaa.* [She reaches out to touch Paro.] She is shaking completely with her eyes on. I can feel she moves. *Ho ho ho ho, mudda dada* little *pusse,* yes. A *gulla* little feel. . . .

Jena takes Paro out of the basket and sets it in Ingrid's lap. She asks if it's too heavy. Ingrid replies, "A bit." Jena adjusts Paro so that it sits more comfortably in Ingrid's lap. The interaction between Paro and Ingrid intensifies as she hugs Paro and rubs its back. The robot begins to respond to Ingrid's touch and her attempts to speak.

> I: Well who says that? [Paro squeals] Huh? [Paro squeals] Who says you must time two times? No one says that, do they? Huh? *pusse lisse.* Yes . . . you are so cute. [Paro squeals twice] You are also *fusse* so much. Yes, yes . . . [Ingrid laughs] Yes, you are. You are a nice seal. [Paro squeals] You have a nice voice. [Paro squeals] *Oh la la. Oh la la,* no. [Paro squeals] It is also. *Oh la la la.* And it is nice. So nice. [Ingrid kisses Paro and laughs] *Pusse birra,* yes. Yes (laughs). It is the little *buller. La la gaka, la la gaka.*

Jena sits next to Ingrid as Ingrid continues to cuddle, rub, and touch Paro. She watches Ingrid kiss Paro and respond to Paro's squeals with phrases and noises of her own. At one point, Jena asks Ingrid if she would like a blanket. Ingrid says yes, and she now sits with furry Paro wrapped in a blanket, as if cradling a child. Jena tries to join in the exchange of sounds and words.

> I: Little *pusse,* how you are feeling good. [Paro squeals] Yes, and *doebbe,* you have been tumbling around. All the time and being sad. Yes . . .

And you have been *kisse* down into it. No you shall not. You must be
a *gop*. Yes. [Paro squeals three times] You are so sucking. They are so
sweet. You must be here, right? And be with the guardian. It is named
Noran? She is named Noran or something?

J: I think so.

I: Don't even know what they are called but it doesn't mean anything
(laughs). *Oooh. Haha.* Yeees. Yeees. *Kaaa yaaaa la la.*

J: Ingrid, do you remember?

I: [ignoring Jena] Yes, ah, yes, then come over. I will come with you.
[Paro squeals] Yes. [Paro squeals] Well don't cry. Don't do that little
honey. Mother is coming. [Paro squeals] There we go. No, don't either.
[Paro squeals] You are blinding. It is you, you *billa* game. Yes, yes, yes
(laughs). No, it was you this time that must *prorororo bop bop bop bop
bop.* Yes, wanted, wanted, wanted. [Paro squeals] *Ay yay yay yay yay
yay.* Yes. [Paro squeals]

The interaction between Paro and Ingrid is so emotionally intense, it is hard
for Jena to engage with Ingrid. Ingrid appears to get more lucid and expressive. Coincidentally, Paro begins to lose power. Jena gently encourages Ingrid
to return Paro back to her basket. (Although this Paro had no name, at points
Ingrid refers to Paro using feminine gender pronouns, so I do here).

I: Little nice *lulla leila kulla. La la la la.* We are not angry with you. We
love you. We do, *buller.* You must remember. [Paro squeals] Ooooh,
no. [Paro squeals twice] Yes, *uh la la uh. Ulllana.* Just forget mother
and say it to them. [kisses Paro] There are sometimes someone. They
don't understand anything, do they? They don't. No. But I am going
home. [Paro squeals] You stick your pieces in no leg. Look at the tail.
[Ingrid hums to herself] Oh dear, you are nice, yes. [Paro squeals]
But I love you. [Paro squeals] I love you, I do. I really do, yes. [Paro
squeals]. It is. Yes, so real and true (laughs). Aren't you happy? Huh?
Have you got mothers that are there? You have what we need to take
care of them . . . ?

J: We can put it in the basket, Ingrid.

I: Yes, something give you.

J: We can put it in the basket if you want.

I: Yes, uh . . .

J: We can put it here to sleep. Shall we do that?

I: Yes. Ooooh . . .

. . .

J: Let's help each other. Come on. Now we lift . . .

I: There, like that. [They lift Paro into the basket together] Yes, like that.
    Yes, now she lies like that. There she lies like that.

J: [Copying Ingrid's gendered speech and mimicking her phrasing] There.
    She lies there.

. . .

I: Is she okay?

J: She is fine there in the basket.

I: Look at her sleep. [begins humming a lullaby]

J: She is so cute.

. . .

I: It's true. She says, too, your mother. She says mother is the best. She is
    the best, right? And she means it.

J: She means it.

I: Right, yes. Now it is done. There it was done.

In her book *Alone Together*, the anthropologist Sherry Turkle reports
being troubled by how interactions between elderly individuals and Paro in
US nursing homes are described. Calling the verbal responses of such individuals to Paro's squeals a "conversation," Turkle tells us, is to "forgot what it
is to have a conversation" (Turkle 2011, 107). Paro, like other sociable robots,
cannot understand human emotion, "cannot care . . . [and] cannot pretend
[to care] because it can only pretend" (Turkle 2011, 124). Turkle's admonition
is worth considering, especially in light of the tendency to anthropomorphize
robots when describing their artificial intelligence systems. Indeed, Paro
cannot converse in an authentically human way. But in watching Danish care
workers work with Paro and in talking with them about the use of Paro,
questions about the authenticity of interactions with Paro emerged much less
frequently than expressions of awe at the impact Paro can have on individuals
with dementia.

This is not to say that care workers never worried about the ethics of
using Paro with older adults. Typically, though, ethical concerns addressed
less the character of interactions with Paro and more its ontological status as
an object. Care workers I met regularly reflected on the ethics of presenting
Paro. Should they tell a person that it's a real seal? Should they instead say

that it's a robot? Uniformly, when they raised this issue, they stated that they always tell a person with dementia that Paro is a robot.[8]

I have excerpted the session with Ingrid, Paro, and Jena at length in part to demonstrate how complicated the ethics of using Paro become in practice. During the session, Jena avoids pointing out that Paro is not a living seal and therefore does not need to sleep. Instead, she actively helps to create a world with Ingrid where Paro is a living thing in need of sleep. At the start, she hedges and refers to Paro with the impersonal "it." But gradually she adopts the pronoun "she" to refer to Paro, just as Ingrid does, and even uses the nonsense word *buller* that Ingrid uses. In so doing, Jena brings herself more deeply into the social space of interaction between Ingrid and Paro. Knowing that Paro's battery is running low, Jena creatively suggests that they make Paro sleep. Ingrid helps Jena do this, and soon they are aligned in the same social world, both commenting on the "sleeping" robot—a moment of connection. Jena knows, of course, that Paro is a robot and that robots do not sleep. She is only behaving *as if* Paro is sleeping because this is the world she is creating with Ingrid. Does Ingrid know that Paro is a robot? Is she, like Jena, behaving *as if* Paro is in need of sleep? Does she think that Paro has suddenly come alive and needs to sleep? It is impossible to know for sure.

For care workers like Jena, issues of the cognitive—what residents under their care really *think* Paro is—are less important than the effect interactions with Paro have on the *affective*; that is, how residents come to *feel* in response to Paro. Shifts in affect lead to changes in behavior and can even, as they do for Ingrid, improve lucidity and mental activity. Mutually creating a world, stepping if only for a moment into a shared social world, was a technique used to cultivate a sense of well-being—a sense of "life quality"—for people with dementia. This *working with* rather than working against to correct, adjust, or modify beliefs and actions was the mark of good care technique, the kind of technique that Thomas Kitwood might advocate. It requires creativity and an openness to experimentation.

After Paro is placed back in the basket, Jena sits back down between me and Ingrid. She turns to me, "When Ingrid sits with Paro, she speaks in a normal way. We can talk together. This effect lasts for several hours. When Paro is not here, she can hardly speak." As if on cue, Ingrid turns to Jena and asks, "So, what are you doing next month?" "I don't really know, Ingrid. It's summer vacation," she replies. "So, you get vacation?" Ingrid inquires further. "Yes, yes," Jena tells her and turns back to me, continuing her previous point, "See, it's very nice because now we can communicate. She doesn't just talk about the things in this room. She can also talk about things happening outside, in the future, ask about other things, even give some feedback." She tells me later that during a recent session with Paro, Ingrid remembered that Jena had recently returned from a trip to China and asked her how it went. There are stuffed animals and dolls in the room as well, some with lipstick and makeup smeared on them. Ingrid occasionally tries to put it on them. Jena uses these with Ingrid as well, but she stresses that they don't "open her up" as much as Paro. Paro "has a stronger effect," Jena tells me, because "Paro responds."

There have been attempts to quantify the physiological effects that Paro has on older adults with dementia.[9] Most are short-term field experiments that measure facial expressions, cortisol levels, or another physiological proxy for stress. In centering the measurement of objective quantities, such studies do not depend on the kind of subjective reports of state of mind typically used in evaluating health-related QoL. They thereby avoid the difficulties of evaluating efficacy for persons with varying ability to speak. Yet, for care workers like Jena, efficacy is rarely framed in such granular terms. Effects are simply big or small, transitory or persistent. They do not just align with gender—men can respond just as positively to the robot, despite the clearly maternal relationships that women, like Ingrid above, commonly establish in sessions. They can also be inconsistent. It is hard to know how a person might react to Paro, even if they have had a positive experience with Paro in the recent past. Generally, however, the more severe the dementia, the better the response to Paro. As one manager of a nursing home put it to me, "Sicker is better. There is a stage of dementia where people are not realistic about their condition—they still think they are normal. And they can get mad at you when you present Paro to them. 'Do you think I'm crazy?' they say. 'I can see it's a toy.' But there is a further stage, where people are not as aware of the progression of their symptoms." Yet, even in these cases, efficacy can vary. Dementia care with Paro is necessarily experimental. The capacity of Paro to sense and respond is key to its value but it is neither assured in practice nor does it arise in isolation. It depends on the facilitation of a skilled care worker who can optimize the robot's functionality *in situ*. In everyday practice, then, caring well with Paro is an iterative process, one that builds on past practices of caring with digital technology.

Redirecting Affect

When interactions with Paro did calm a person or change their mood, care workers rarely spoke of affective change as being an end in itself. The well-being of individual residents may be the professed objective of Kitwoodian dementia care, but achieving well-being in practice also helps staff complete challenging tasks associated with the care of individual persons. What's more, it assists in the perhaps even more difficult task of managing a residential community of people with dementia. On the individual level, positive affect helps maintain personal hygiene; on the level of the institution, it promotes the safety of staff and residents.

Here again the sociotechnical assemblage of Jena, Ingrid, and Paro is instructive. Jena tells me,

> Sometimes when I visit Ingrid, she is very, very angry, and we can't communicate at all. She'll just slam the door on me . . . Or sometimes when we are going to help Ingrid in the bathroom—she needs a diaper change or something—she will fight because she can't understand what we're trying to do. So, if it smells in here when I come in, sometimes I can go get Paro and sit here for 10–15 minutes with Ingrid. When we put Paro to sleep, we can go to the bathroom, take a bath, change clothes, get ready for bed, wash the dining table, or whatever, and it's no problem.

As much as the achievement of psychological well-being is the objective of dementia care in Denmark, care workers still need to make sure that the physical needs of residents are satisfied. They need to be fed and bathed, have their teeth brushed, and kept clean from urine and feces to prevent infection. The behavioral symptoms of dementia, like the anger and noncompliance reported by Jena, can frustrate the efforts of staff to keep residents nourished and clean. In a previous era, the need to satisfy the physical needs of residents might have taken precedence. Care staff might have taken coercive action in the interest of ensuring physical safety and health. Today, however, working with a noncompliant resident to create an environment comfortable enough that care tasks could be performed was the preferred course of action. As Jena describes above, to open a path toward social engagement and the support of Ingrid's physiological needs, she uses Paro as a tool to help Ingrid calm down enough that Jena's work can proceed. Feeling the machine (Paro) helps stem emotional distress and facilitate the satisfaction of physical needs.

Expressions of anger and aggression most concerned staff and inspired hope for a successful intervention with Paro. Angry and aggressive residents cannot only make care difficult; they can also threaten the health and safety of others. For some citizens, like Ingrid, daily engagement with Paro helped manage the expression of negative affect in an ongoing way. For others, anger and aggression can erupt unpredictably. In such cases, staff typically first try distraction. While I was talking with one nursing home director, for example, I noticed a box of nerf balls near her desk. I asked her what they were for, and she told me, "We've learned to have some of these on hand. Sometimes one of the male residents down there [she gestures toward the dementia-care ward] gets quite aggressive and comes after people. When that happens, we throw the balls at him. Just to distract him. He says, 'whoa, whoa, whoa,' and then we can get out of the way, or he gets distracted and forgets why he was angry in the first place." Obviously, Paro is too expensive to throw at people, but the interest in distracting people from their anger lent it value. The director of another nursing home told me, "When I have a person who is very restless, who wants to leave the nursing home, who cannot get calm because there is too much disquiet in him [she uses the masculine gender], and he's starting to be maybe aggressive or angry, then I will think: How can I help this person by making a better life for him. And then that is where the seal comes in . . . so he forgets his bad mood."

The utility of Paro as a technology of distraction to reduce or otherwise redirect aggression often came up in response to questions about its cost. Aside from its ability to better the QoL of individual patients, justifications of Paro's price (the equivalent of several thousand US dollars) were made based on its potential to reduce the time staff needed to handle difficult patients or avoid the loss of staff time resulting from injury. The director of a nursing home outside of Copenhagen put it to me like this: "We have an older man, he is . . . he is very stuck, and can't do anything for himself . . . We have to take a walk with him each day for about one hour to calm him down. I have to think about priorities. Is it better for me to take him out for a walk so in the evening when there's only two caretakers down there, he'll be calm? That's also my philosophy with Paro. If I invest some money, I can avoid aggressive situations where some of the caretakers get hurt." She then told me of one woman who injured two of her care workers, directly and indirectly:

> I have two employees who are on sick leave. There is one woman who is very aggressive and can hit people. She hit one of the care workers who

had come into her room to help her. She got hurt and then took additional leave to deal with post-traumatic stress. The other tried to avoid being hit and injured her knee. It's very expensive for me to have workers out on sick leave for a long time. If I can avoid these situations, spending 35,000–40,000 kroner ($5,500–6,000) on a Paro is a good investment.

These sentiments were echoed by a director for welfare services in the municipality of Lejre on the outskirts of Copenhagen. "If there is a person who is violent because they don't know what's going on around them, then that person is going to be violent toward me. If Paro can help this person not be violent but to be present in the moment, then that's a success." Anne, the nursing home director from Køge, added, "If we work well together, we can bring some life quality to the elderly . . . When I first asked [municipal authorities] for a Paro, my hope was that it could be used to give patients some quality time and to help them be calm, especially the aggressive ones."

It was not just managers who are concerned about violence. Two care workers at a nursing home in Copenhagen spoke with me after they concluded a "Wellness Session" with four residents. The Wellness Session was designed with prevention in mind, an attempt to keep residents calm and docile. The two care workers, Tine and Andrea, put the residents into a circle, then turned on soft ambient music, started up a diffuser with an aromatherapy scent, and laid red blankets on the laps of the residents. They reclined the wheelchairs and circulated among the residents, giving them head and face massages and encouraging them to relax. They also passed two Paro robots among the residents, letting them cuddle and pet Paro for a while until they moved onto another person in the group. The entire session was considered part of an ongoing plan to maintain a sedate environment in the nursing home. Touch—the touch of the care workers on the residents, the touch of the residents on Paro, the feeling of Paro in their laps, whimpering and occasionally kicking—structured the session. Still, for one woman who sat some distance away on a couch looking out a window toward the courtyard, tactile interaction was not possible. "We can't touch her," Tine and Andrea told me. "She gets upset and she gets aggressive. So, we can't give her massages." For this woman, Paro became an important mediator. "[Sitting on the couch], she gets some energy, some warmth, some sun. She'll look at Paro . . . You can't help it, I mean you see those eyes . . . We can't touch her, but we can see her face, how she reacts. And then we can figure out our next move."

Used creatively, Paro helps these women reduce the potential for aggression in residents under their care, lessening the possibility that stress will build up to violence and even affording some insight into state of mind.

I observed a similar application of Paro as a mediator at a nursing home in a northwestern suburb of Copenhagen. At this site, Anders, a male helper at the facility, eagerly showed me the notebook in which he and his coworkers tracked their sessions with Paro. He told me that they had found their Paro, whom they called "Luffe" ("big glove"), useful as a tool to distract "older men who get aggressive." For women, he told me, Paro often elicits a "caring impulse." While there were some men who responded similarly, he emphasized how Paro could help deflect anger in other men. Anders led me out of the room where we had been talking toward another. As we approached, his walking pace slowed. His body stiffened and his face tensed up. He put a finger to his lips and whispered, "This is a very dangerous man." I could see no one around, but he gestured inside the room. "We have to be very careful. He can try to hit." He announced our entry and led me slowly into the room. The man was sitting on a couch next to his wife, who happened to be visiting that day. Anders knelt down to the same level as the seated man. He began gently petting Paro and gingerly extended his arms out toward him, trying to gauge his interest. The man didn't seem particularly interested in Luffe but he didn't react aggressively either. Luffe physically mediated the interaction between Anders and the man. The robot became an object of interest that also kept safe distance between him and the man. Anders sat down in a chair, still holding and petting Luffe. He spoke for a few more minutes with the man's wife, who asked several questions about the robot. Seeing that the man had no interest in engaging with Luffe, however, Anders said goodbye and walked with me out of the room.

The tactical use of distraction employed by care workers to defuse violent disruption makes visible social norms that extend beyond enhancement of individual QoL or the novel use of the robot Paro. Care professionals I met were reluctant to coerce any resident to do things against their will, even in the interest of physical health, or to restrain outbursts of anger or aggression with physical force. This stemmed not just from a commitment to the philosophy of Tom Kitwood. Care workers operate within a legal context that holds a person's right to self-determination paramount and strictly regulates the use of coercive force on persons who are in institutional care.

In the facilities I visited, staff told me proudly that citizens in their care maintained their own rooms (apartments) within the nursing home. They could decorate these rooms to their liking—most outfitted their rooms with objects from their former homes—and they could control access to them with lock and key. Care workers had to ask to enter individual rooms. Doors in and out of nursing homes were never locked, and residents with dementia were permitted free entry and exit. They could not, except for very rare cases, be forcibly confined since such confinement would violate the right to self-determination. Similarly, forcing a resident to take a bath or to have their diaper changed, for example, could occur only *after* care workers had tried to persuade the resident of its necessity for at least five hours. Once five hours passed, care workers could take action that they believed would be in the best interest of a resident's hygiene or safety. Coercive action had to be communicated in writing to supervisors (usually the director of the nursing home), who would then forward reports to municipal authorities. Subsequently, a dementia professional counselor (*Demensfagligrådgiver*, or DPC), would visit the nursing home to interview the supervisor who talked with the care worker. The DPC would review the case and evaluate whether the action was necessary from a health perspective. The report would then be sent to a legal authority at the municipal office to determine whether the action was legal. If determined to be legal, then the oversight process would end. If not, the nursing home would be notified and directed to engage staff in additional training in the avoidance of force.

Suffice to say, managers and workers both worked to avoid the use of force given the labor-intensive reporting required after such events occur. Working with residents rather than pushing against their will, even in the interest of health or safety, derives from more than just theories of person-centered care. Working with residents keeps care workers and nursing homes within the bounds of the law. Accordingly, patients who are angry, disruptive, or otherwise violent pose a problem for institutions where coercive action is so tightly circumscribed. Nursing homes have an interest in modulating the affect of residents. Modulating negative affect and avoiding the use of force is in their best interest. For these reasons, Paro's utility in changing negative affect to positive affect lent it significant value in the eyes of Danish care workers.

Caring Infrastructure

Paro is not the only technology of affect modulation in Danish nursing homes. Subtle manipulation of behavior is literally inscribed on the walls of nursing homes themselves. This became apparent on a visit to a nursing home in the municipality of Lejre. After talking with staff there about plans for introducing Paro to residents, I was led through the facility by Lena, a nurse. At the end of one hallway, I saw a brightly colored floor-to-ceiling painting of an outdoor scene. It was done in broad strokes of bright blue, green, and white, and depicted trees, grass, and a cloud-filled sky. At the center were two red birds facing toward each other, so close that it looked like they were kissing, if birds could kiss (see figure 4.1). As we drew closer, I saw that I was looking at a painting on a double door. The beaks of the two birds met right at the doorknob.

"You don't touch birds," Lena told me. "If a person with dementia wants to get out, they might start looking for a door." But they would be reluctant to reach for this door handle, if it meant touching birds. The birds were meant to provide a distraction so that the person would, ideally, forget that they had the urge to look for a door in the first place. Creatively masking interior structures enlisted those very structures in the care of residents housed inside them. The door-in-disguise functioned much like the nerf balls that Anne described throwing at agitated residents to distract them from their agitation. The painting effectively changed an exit into an enclosure for those without the cognitive capacity to distinguish actual birds from painted birds. Those who recognized the painting would, presumably, have sufficient mental capacity to leave without endangering themselves. The desire to go outside would shift in line with the interest of the nursing home in keeping them inside. By strategically employing "dementia-friendly design" staff could subtly influence the behavior of residents by working with, arguably even exploiting, their cognitive limitations.

One nursing home I visited had created a sort of triage system. On a door leading out from the interior of the facility to the lobby, they had painted a bright white picket fence. The painting stretched across the door frame to cover the entire wall, with the top of the painted fence crossing just under the door knob. The fence lacked any identifiable gate. Staff showing me around the facility made clear that the painting was meant to create the illusion of enclosure. "You don't ever try to walk through a fence, do you?" As we passed

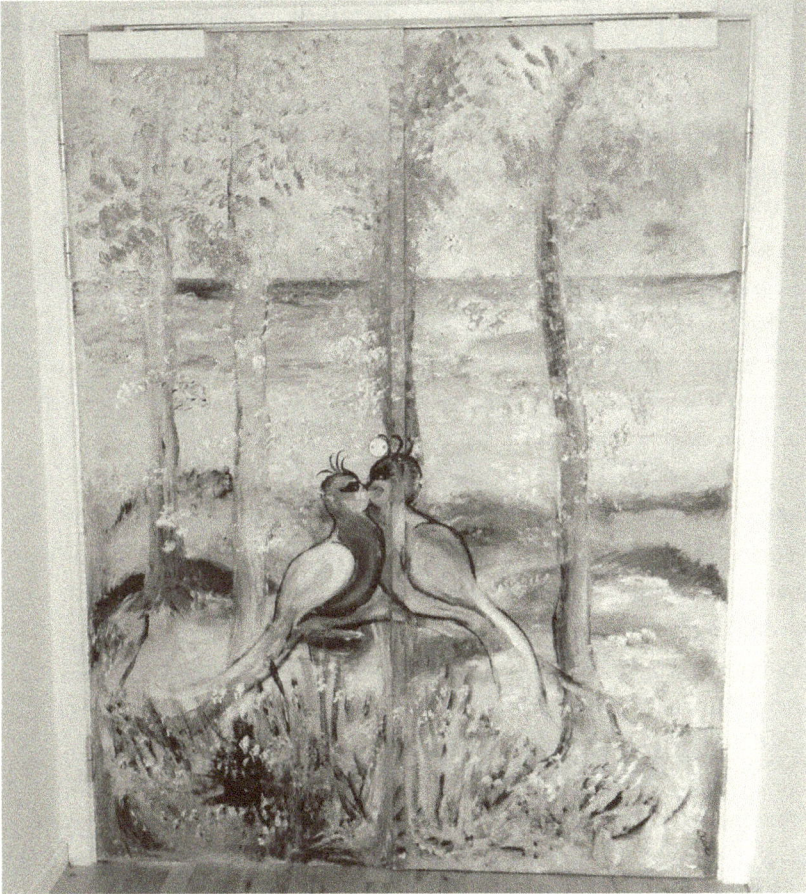

FIGURE 4.1 Infrastructures of Care.   Creatively masking unlocked exit doors helps to keep residents with dementia inside Danish nursing homes without forcibly confining them. Photo by author.

through the door, we entered a long vestibule at the end of which was another door. To open this door, one had to push an unmarked button on the wall about fifteen feet in front of it. Past that door, in the lobby atrium, were several floor-to-ceiling windows that looked out on a wooden cage containing live birds. The birds were a last line of defense. Should a resident make it past the painted fence, push the button on the wall, and enter the lobby, the hope was that they might get distracted by the birds in the cage and forget about leaving the facility.

I thought that I had encountered an exception to this trend on a visit to a brand-new nursing home in Copenhagen. The nursing home looked like a typical apartment complex: brightly white walls, lightly stained natural wood floors, thick leather sitting chairs, automated entry doors, a mounted flat-screen TV, and decorative lamps made out of artfully twisted plastic. "Yes, the lamps." Janet, an administrator at the facility, told me with a roll of the eyes. "The designer really wanted to have nice lamps." While sumptuously decorated, the facility did not meet some fundamental needs of the persons with dementia who lived there. Staff had to repaint lounges so that colors contrasted enough for people with dementia, who might not be able to differentiate a chair from a wall. They coated the walls of hallways in bright yellow, so that residents could more easily identify the white doors to their rooms.

Other doors in the facility were purposely hidden. When Janet took me up to a floor for residents with advanced cases of dementia, she noted that exit doors were painted the same white color as the hallway. Rather than disguise the door as an outdoor scene like the nursing home in Lejre, the use of color made it hard for occupants of the floor to distinguish door from wall. The doors also had two latches; one at waist-height, the other at eye level. To open them, one had to push down on the lower latch and up on the higher latch simultaneously.

"How odd, then," I thought to myself as I set out at the end of my visit, "that they would have automatic doors at the entrance to the facility." As if on cue, I found myself standing at these very doors, unable to exit. I paced back and forth in confusion trying to get the doors to open. Soon, a staff member passing by sensed my distress and pointed to two white switches mounted on the door frame to my left. The left switch had an arrow pointing down on it; the right switch, an arrow pointing up. Pushing the bottom of the left switch and the top of the right switch activated the doors. "We have people with dementia here so we have this device," she told me as I exited sheepishly.

These examples indicate that Paro is not the only material technology brought to bear on the care of people with dementia in Danish nursing homes. Strategically decorated interior surfaces, cleverly concealed door switches, intellectually demanding locks, even nerf balls, stuffed dolls, wellness sessions, "sensory-integration" rooms *(snoezelen)*, basement areas converted into shopping streets with functioning cafes, general stores, and bars, courtyard "dementia gardens" with edible plants, all are enlisted in subtly manipulating the feelings of residents with dementia. This is why care workers I met,

from Olivia to others, described Paro as "one more tool" to use in the care
of dementia, though many admired its effectiveness. In fact, unless a miracle
cure is someday discovered, variation in the expression of dementia symptoms
make it unlikely that any single technology will ever be the *only* way to care
for dementia. In Denmark, Paro works together with the physical architecture of nursing homes to redirect the affect of residents with dementia while
respecting their rights to self-determination.

Encoding Care

Paro may be just one more tool, but the effect of emotionally intense interactions with the robot reaches far beyond the walls of nursing homes and the
borders of Denmark. Engagement with the robot in Denmark cycles back into
the development, marketing, and promotion of the device in Japan, much like
the "data selves" of elderly residents in Japan travel beyond the nursing homes
through essays and presentations by the Robot Therapy Group. This came
through clearly in a presentation Dr. Shibata gave to a group of Japanese
roboticists in June 2011 that I attended. The presentation began in Japan with
a familiar review of the aging-society-as-problem and care-robots-as-solution,
particularly the contribution that Paro could make to dementia care. Dr. Shibata spoke of a woman in a nursing home who often roamed the hallways of
her nursing home and a man who often looked uneasy and screamed when he
felt uncomfortable. Both calmed down after "feeling" *(fureau)* Paro, he said,
based on EEG measurements taken before and after. Shibata then pivoted
quickly to Denmark. He discussed the Be Safe Project, field tests of Paro,
and the decision of municipalities to invest in Paro. He beamed when an-
nouncing Paro's adoption by 150 nursing homes and orders for one thousand
more, but he stressed that Danish authorities require a person to be certified
before using Paro in practice. This certification course, he added, introduces
Paro's technological features along with effective "ways of deploying [Paro]
in practice."

Mention of the certification course marked a key moment in the presentation. Dr. Shibata had emphasized Paro's strengths as a technology, but the
required course suggested that Paro could not operate effectively without a
skilled human facilitator. As if to return the discussion to the technological,
he noted how close supervision in Denmark contributed to the improvement
of Paro: "In Denmark, they don't just get a certificate, start using Paro, and

then stop. They keep records about how and for whom Paro worked well. Until now, they've held four 'Paro User' conferences where care workers present and share information. Afterwards, they send all that data to me. We use that data as the basis on which to improve Paro going forward." Additional certification courses were planned for other European countries and the United States. In light of this, Dr. Shibata continued, his company planned to release a manual for care workers.

Dr. Shibata's presentation seemed well rehearsed, and mention of the manual furnished proof. Dr. Shibata and his team had already written, tested, and published a manual for care worker's the previous year, in collaboration with academics at Tokyo Metropolitan University. In English, the text is called *Caregiver's Manual for Robot Therapy: Practical Use of Therapeutic Seal Robot Paro in Elderly Facilities* (Wada and Inoue 2010).[10] There is no suggestion in the *Manual* that Paro be left for elderly individuals in facilities to interact with on their own. In fact, the *Manual* recommends that facilities "assign a Paro handler to intervene in the therapy and facilitate it as required" (Wada and Inoue 2010, 7). Illustrations of interactions with Paro show at least one care worker (always a woman dressed in an apron) and at least one person, either care worker or person with dementia, touching Paro. Discussion of the symptoms of dementia and person-centered care are not referenced directly in the *Manual*. But the attention given to introducing Paro, guiding interactions with it, and withdrawing the robot carefully and with respect for the individual life experience of the patients parallels the approach taken in the Danish certification course, with particular reference to people with dementia (Wada and Inoue 2010, 7–14). One of Dr. Shibata's colleagues, who was himself involved in designing and testing the *Manual* in Japan, told me, in an interview in June 2011, that it emerged out of a perceived need to improve how Paro is used within facilities.

> The effect of Paro changes depending on the care worker who uses it. The reason why we created a manual is because there are two types of carers: those who naturally know how to handle *(atsukaeru)* Paro effectively without special instruction and those who don't. People who have a natural ability to handle Paro well have a difficult time explaining how they do it to people who don't. If we hadn't created a reference manual, then these people would forever have trouble handling Paro well.

Dr. Shibata and his colleague recognize the role that care workers play in enhancing Paro's effectiveness in practice. The assemblage of Paro–care worker–care recipient is also vital to "improving" *(kairyō)* the functionality of the device itself. Developers seek advice about how to iterate their device from people who use it effectively; users make more effective use of a device that is better suited to their needs. Innovation does not proceed only in line with the imagination of a technologist. Through iterative engagement, caring for people with robots is entangled with the making of care robots.

In 2013, two years after Dr. Shibata's lecture and my conversation with his colleague, Shibata's venture firm, Intelligent Systems, along with his laboratory at the National Institute of Advanced Industrial Science and Technology, released a ninth-generation Paro. This version marked the first major iteration of the robot since 2004, right around when Olivia remembers first seeing Paro in Denmark. In a press release, just after introducing the name of the product, the company notes that Paro is used in therapy for people with dementia, cognitive disabilities, and developmental disabilities in over 70 percent of Danish municipalities (Intelligent Systems Co. 2013, 1). The company writes further, "In collaboration with DTI (Danish Technological Institute), AIST conducted joint research and development and sponsored four 'user conferences' *(yūza kaigi)* in Denmark. AIST also sponsored three research conferences on robot therapy with Paro in Japan. *Primarily on the basis of feedback from users at these conferences, we made improvements to Paro's hardware and software*" (Intelligent Systems Co. 2013, 1, my emphasis). The Japanese research conferences to which the press release refers began in September 2012, one year before the ninth-generation Paro was released. The first three conference speakers were from Denmark, in addition to presentations by Dr. Shibata and his colleagues in Japan. Given the Danish presence, it is hard to distinguish these conferences on the basis of location alone (see http://intelligent-system.jp).[11]

In terms of improvements, the company upgraded the speed of Paro's CPU, extended its battery life, strengthened its mechanical frame, and enhanced the hygienic properties of its fur. They also added brown, cherry, and charcoal fur colors to existing white and gold. But the key modification made to the robot would likely go unnoticed by users. For the first time, Intelligent Systems segmented Paro into two devices: one for use in therapy *(serapii-yō)*; another designed for the robot's original role as a pet substitute *(petto-yō).* The two models are exactly the same on the inside and outside. The nature of their operating code is what separates them. For the therapy version, Paro's behavior-selection algorithms *(kōdō seisei arugorizumu)* are optimized to "maximize therapeutic efficacy and enhance ease-of-use by care workers" (Intelligent Systems Co. 2013, 2). Exactly how the algorithm has been modified is left unspecified and is likely proprietary anyway. What is clear is that Paro's feedback effect—its impact on the affect of persons with dementia in Danish nursing homes—has been encoded into the robot itself, in an effort to generate even more intense feedback than before.

"The problem with Paro is that there's been no new version *(bāshon-appu ga nai)*. It's much the same as it was years ago. They only tweaked the algorithm. No wonder it hasn't done better in Japan," a young member of the Robot Therapy Group told me as we spoke over drinks after concluding a therapy session. The engineer bore no ill will toward Dr. Shibata or his robot (even though, as I noted in the previous chapter, the group made only incidental use of Paro in its sessions). His comment came in response to my asking why he and others at our table thought that Paro had not been received as enthusiastically in Japanese dementia care as it had elsewhere. Perhaps reflecting an engineering bias, he and others at the table traced the problem to a lack of new features; a failure, that is, to iterate Paro fast enough to both keep up with existing demand and generate yet more. Dr. Shibata and colleagues were doing all the right things. They were continually gathering data about Paro's effectiveness, both in their own research projects and at user and research conferences. But, in the eyes of these roboticists, they had failed to convert those insights quickly enough into innovation. Salesmanship had trumped engineering. "He [Dr. Shibata] is spending his time traveling the world to sell Paro, and not enough time improving it," he said. I countered that Paro seemed to have done well in Denmark. He threw up his hands. "He's always talking about Denmark. Where else has Paro done well?"

Dr. Shibata and his collaborators typically attribute Paro's lack of appeal in Japan to the "group orientation" of Japanese eldercare facilities. Nursing homes in Japan, they say, tend not to make investments in devices unless everyone in the facility benefits from them. In Denmark, by contrast, if a device is used only by a small portion of a nursing home population, facilities will still consider an investment in the device. Shibata often attributes this to the influence of Kitwoodian person-centered care models on Danish dementia care, especially the importance it places on understanding patients as individuals. Wherever this philosophy spreads (e.g., other European countries, increasingly the United States), he implies, Paro is likely to be successfully adopted. Something that goes unmentioned is the issue of public financing. Despite the support of Paro's early development by Japanese government bodies (AIST, NEDO), Paro is not eligible for reimbursement under Japan's LTCI.[12] Without subsidies, individuals or institutions have to bear the full cost of purchasing Paro (roughly $3,500 in 2017, not including additional maintenance plans), a clear disincentive for care facilities that have little budget room for such a significant investment.

Hearing the engineer's words brought to mind a conversation I had a few months prior with Olivia, the woman who was primarily responsible for introducing Paro into Danish dementia care. Olivia agreed that Paro had been something of a sensation when it first came to Denmark in the early 2000s. Paro helped to change public attitudes toward robots and related digital technologies of care from negative to positive. As Dr. Shibata put it in the 2011 lecture I attended, Paro was an "icebreaker" that opened the field of care up to other kinds of digital technologies. Indeed, a Danish gloss on these kinds of technologies, "welfare technology" *(velfærdsteknologi)*, emerged in the wake of Paro's introduction in 2007.

Yet, by the time we spoke in 2017, Olivia's organization, the Danish Technological Institute, had stopped distributing Paro. Paro had matured beyond the emerging technologies that the firm usually handles. It was now sold by a company called Gloria Municare—"selling more slowly," Olivia cautioned, "than it did with us in the beginning." I asked if she thought this was because the market was saturated. "I think there are many different reasons. One is that many got the Paro they needed. Now you even see that many Paro are asleep and covered up [in disuse], but I wouldn't say the market is saturated. In my opinion, you should have a Paro in every nursing home, as one tool. But it might be too much for a home with just thirty residents to have an expensive tool like this."

She continued:

But what has also happened in the last six years or so is that many other innovative welfare technologies have attracted attention and are being implemented, so the focus is not just on Paro. The focus is on welfare technologies in general. Paro still has a special position. Everyone knows Paro. If you take a taxi, you should ask the driver if they've heard of Paro. "Sure, that's the white baby harp seal," they'll say. Paro is still well known but it doesn't have a unique position anymore . . . Shibata has a new version now, with a new battery and weight. But he is pressed by other products. There are cats and teddy bears. Some have warm stomachs. Some make nice sounds as well. There are now many products in the category. Sure, they're not as intelligent [as Paro], but maybe intelligence isn't that important?

Instead of more computing power, Olivia, like most care workers with whom I spoke in Denmark, longed for a simple but technically impossible feature: fur that is easy to remove and clean. People with dementia often try to feed or apply makeup to Paro. But the only way to clean the robot is to send it back to company headquarters in Japan. Care workers would prefer to do this themselves. However, it is not possible to make a Paro that is easier to clean without fundamentally changing its features, since Paro's sensors are tightly integrated into its fur. Despite its many upgrades, care workers do not really want a Paro that is smarter, more responsive, or even longer lasting. Its durability and ease-of-use are what continue to make it attractive relative to other competing technologies.

These views from Japan and Denmark suggest that Paro's technological future is uncertain. As enthusiasm for the device wanes in Denmark, it is unclear what kind of user feedback will drive Paro's innovation. (Olivia noted that Paro-user conferences in Denmark stopped around 2011 because so much of the feedback they got replicated what they had learned previously.) Still, Paro remains a landmark product in Denmark and in Japan. Paro demonstrated how the skillful use of robotics technology could enhance QoL for people with dementia. It illustrated how activities of care can be integrated into the feedback cycles that guide innovation. At the same time, perhaps, it revealed the limitations of iterative engagements of care: they may not lead quickly enough to continued innovation (i.e., the gap between eight- and ninth-generation Paro) or may drive innovation in the wrong direction (e.g., improving AI instead of cleanable fur). An attempt to close that gap with faster, digitally connected technologies is in part the aim of another care robot from Japan called HAL, an exoskeleton for physical therapy that I examine in the next chapter.

FIVE

Engaging HAL

Jenny stands on a treadmill, her torso wrapped in a support harness and her eyes fixed on a full-length mirror in front of her. Her shoulders are square and taut. Her lips are drawn together in concentration. Her fingers curl around support handrails. She takes a deep breath, exhaling just as the rubber belt beneath her whirs into action. Now she walks, not as smoothly as she once did but with more assurance, more fluidity, and more dexterity than usual. She studies herself in the mirror. Her focused expression relaxes into a smile.

Jenny is not walking alone. Fastened around her waist and running down the sides of her legs is a HAL exoskeleton. Wires snaking out from the exoskeleton attach to Jenny's skin. Their electrodes detect faint electrical impulses traveling along nerve pathways between her brain and legs. In an instant, HAL converts these impulses into digital information. This information is transmitted to a processing unit that, only milliseconds later, activates motors in the joints that provide finely calibrated torque to help Jenny move as she intends. Walking unassisted on a treadmill, or anywhere else for that matter, is not something that Jenny can normally do. She is partially paralyzed from the waist down. Without HAL, Jenny's legs don't work like they used to. Without a body to sense, HAL doesn't work at all.

Jenny is one of several dozen patients who come to Cyberdyne Care Robotics (CCR) in Bochum, Germany, for sessions with the exoskeleton. Most have experienced a traumatic injury to the spine that has impaired their ability to walk; others have gradually lost some walking ability due to stroke or neuromuscular disease. In 2015, CCR remained the only place in the world where patients could undergo medically supervised "Neurorobotic Movement Training" with HAL that is covered by insurance. Not even in Japan, where HAL technology was first invented and developed, could patients access such services.

"Go! Go! Right! Left! Forward!" a therapist, dressed in a gray top and white pants, calls out from behind Jenny. She holds a plastic module that slots into HAL's waistband. On its front, a small LED screen displays real-time visualizations of the pressure Jenny places on her feet, the bend of her knee, and the power provided by the exoskeleton. The therapist can use this information to make adjustments on the fly if needed, but everything is running smoothly now. Half a world away in Japan at Cyberdyne, the maker of HAL, a computer logs the digital traces of Jenny's training session, also in real time.

The therapist slides the module back into the exoskeleton. Beads of sweat have begun to form on Jenny's forehead. She struggles to push her legs forward, urged on by her therapist. This is no leisurely stroll; this is *training*—the term staff at CCR use for these HAL-supported sessions at the facility. Jenny's therapist ducks underneath a support handrail and grabs a metal rod between the exoskeleton's shoe and the end of its plastic leg. She helps Jenny push her leg to full extension—Jenny, therapist, HAL, all work in unison. "Right leg! Right leg!" she yells, encouraging her to keep walking, to keep her legs moving, again and again.

The therapist senses fatigue. It's time to stop for the day. She turns off the treadmill and powers down the HAL suit. She helps Jenny, now released from the harness but still attached to the exoskeleton, settle into a wheelchair. Jenny sips a glass of water and jokes with a team of therapists who now move with the agility of a pit crew as they swiftly unhook her from the machine. Once untethered, Jenny is wheeled down a ramp into an adjoining room. She is helped out of the wheelchair onto a bed where two staff members remove electrodes still stuck to her skin. Two therapists fetch her arm braces and guide her to the starting line of a short-distance track at the center of the room. One pushes record on a video camera mounted on a tripod next to the track, while the other helps Jenny down a ten-meter section. Jenny completes this ten-meter walk before and after each session with HAL. Therapists score her performance (e.g., how far she goes, how much assistance she needs) numerically along a standard Walking Index for Spinal Cord Injury II (WISCI II) scale. Staff at CCR use WISCI-II tests to track improvements in Jenny's walking ability after training with HAL. Sports scientists at CCR, in collaboration with doctors at neighboring Bergmannsheil Hospital, aggregate and analyze such test data for research studies on the efficacy of training with HAL. Poster-sized printouts of article title pages hang prominently around the room. Jenny is just one of many individuals in Germany whose efforts help demonstrate the utility of the exoskeleton from Japan.

For now, she is done for the day. A friend arrives to pick her up. She waves goodbye to the assembled therapists and rides out into a bright summer day.

———

Most of the patients whom I met on visits to CCR in 2015 and 2017 had, like Jenny, experienced traumatic injury. Unlike the residents of nursing homes in Japan and Denmark, they were young, otherwise healthy, and lived mostly independent lives. They came to CCR because they had exhausted the capacity of conventional therapies to help them heal, but they knew that they would never move as fluidly as they once did. This is what doctors have told them and what they have come to accept. Yet they arrive at CCR with the expectation that training with "the robot," as they call HAL, might help them move more, incrementally so, in the future. Neither they nor their therapists or doctors know how much more. There is no way to tell in advance, and no way to know whether they have reached the limit of recovered physical function, short of complete rehabilitation, even after months of dedicated training. The kind of care they seek at CCR is, then, not curative; it is iterative. Even modest recovery of functional mobility is a stimulus to strive for more. Patients at CCR aspire for an optimized, more functional future self.

In this chapter, I examine iterative engagements of care with HAL at CCR and the "affective atmosphere" (Anderson 2009) of aspiration that suffuses it. Hybrid encounters of human patients and robotic exoskeletons are the focus of activity at CCR. But the aspirations that drive those encounters are not limited to patients alone. Therapists who facilitate HAL training are motivated by the chance to use the cutting-edge technology of HAL in new ways to push the recovery of functional mobility beyond what is achievable with conventional techniques. Doctors and sports scientists, working in collaboration with therapists and patients, strive to understand the therapeutic

benefits of HAL technology through research studies and in clinical practice. The outcomes of these studies feed back to therapists to more precisely
inform their approach to patient care. They feed forward in the hands of
business managers toward the expansion of HAL training to new categories
of potential patients. The aspiration of patients for a maximally functional
self similarly parallels the efforts of engineers in Japan who work to improve
the functionality of the HAL exoskeleton based in part on data from actual
training sessions with HAL. As patients work to transform their bodies with
HAL, they contribute to the development of HAL technology. Iterative engagements of care at CCR, then, entangle patients, therapists, doctors, and
managers in Germany with technologists in Japan.

Care in this iterative modality, with aspiration at its center, is what distinguishes CCR from nursing homes in Japan and Denmark. The inexorable
nature of a disease like dementia means that robot-assisted care can only
help minimize the everyday stress of institutional care. AIBO and Paro help
modulate the affect of residents who might be agitated or withdrawn. HAL
similarly responds to the feelings of human wearers—their urge to move,
their wish to walk. Yet, despite the lingering presence of irreparable injury,
patients who train with HAL *can* get better. Their bodies remain optimiz-
able, their brains moldable like plastic. Feedback loops connecting body to
machine and brain to limb do more than channel aspiration and drive the
cyborg body. The very *plasticity* of the brain—its capacity to reorganize itself
in response to new demands on the body—makes possible the incremental
achievement of physical function. At CCR, feedback and response become
the basis of healing, the means of molding a self 2.0.

Loop One: HAL

Overlapping loops of feedback propel the machine that drives activity at
CCR. HAL itself is composed of two control systems—a voluntary control system *(zuii seigyō shisutemu)* and an autonomous control system *(jir-
itsu seigyo shistemu)*—that respond to the intended movement of a human
wearer. The voluntary control system senses electrical traces produced by
nerve signals traveling along motor neuron pathways between the brain and
extremities. It converts these analog impulses into digital data and sends
this data to a central processing unit (CPU) that calculates the trajectory of
an intended movement. Within fractions of a second, before muscles twitch,

a CPU triggers actuators in the upper and middle joints of the exoskeleton that support that intended movement. This voluntary control system works best if there are no interruptions in the motor neuron pathways of the body. The autonomous control system activates when injury has weakened the impulses carried by motor neurons muscles or the wearer's limbs have atrophied significantly. It continuously monitors actual physical movement—shifts in weight from heel to toe, changes in the angular velocity of hip and knee—and provides powered support based on an estimate of the intended trajectory. HAL's developers call the coordinated interaction of these control systems "hybrid assistance." This is what lends the machine its name—"Hybrid Assistive Limb," or HAL.[1] (Fans of science fiction will recognize the tongue-in-cheek nod to the killer AI of the same name in Stanley Kubrick's fiction 1968 film, *2001: A Space Odyssey*.)

Hybrid assistance only works when HAL is connected to a human body. Once attached to HAL, the human body becomes part of a "closed loop of feedback" by which the robot—or, more precisely the human–robot assemblage—operates. Ideally, there is no perceptible lag between the movement of a limb and the movement of the HAL robot suit. HAL thereby pushes the feedback effect of interaction with care robots beyond Paro or AIBO into the unconscious. As a Japanese engineer involved in HAL's development put it to me in 2010, "When you try to move, you move the robot and the robot moves you."[2] The ambiguity of agency in this statement is purposeful. When you move the robot and the robot moves you, you consciously recognize that you and the robot have moved. However, HAL's developers believe that, at an unconscious level, signals are sent back to the brain from the peripheral nervous system, a process the engineer called "interactive biofeedback." Through conscious and unconscious loops of feedback, he continued, eyebrows raised in excitement, HAL technology "finally achieves the fusion of human and robot."

The technology underlying HAL has been in development for over two decades in Japan under the leadership of Yoshiyuki Sankai, a professor of engineering based at the University of Tsukuba. In 2004, Prof. Sankai launched a venture firm, Cyberdyne Corporation, to commercialize his invention. (Another tongue-in-cheek nod: Cyberdyne Systems is the company that makes killer cyborgs in the *Terminator* film franchise.) The technology of hybrid assistance has stayed consistent through the many iterations of HAL technology. Understandings of its potential applications have varied, however.

In 2000, Sankai and his collaborators wrote that HAL-1 aims "to realize the walking aid *and rehabilitation* for . . . person[s] with walking disabilities" (Sankai et al. 2000, 269, my emphasis).[3] The reference to rehabilitation notwithstanding, HAL is framed in this and other publications primarily as a potential mobility aid for frail adults and persons with disabilities.[4] After 2005, HAL is increasingly presented as a potential technological solution for the attendant problems of Japan's aging society, though not necessarily for the use of the aged themselves (Hornyak 2007; Toyoda 2010). In fall 2010, HAL was included as one of four care robots in the Kanagawa Prefecture's Care Robot Promotion Project, a project focused specifically on the care needs of an aging population (see chapter 2). Discursive emphasis on the contribution that HAL technology could make in an aging society continued through the decade.[5] It is no surprise that I was so often referred to HAL during my fieldwork on care robots in Japan from 2009–11.

When I interviewed Prof. Sankai at Cyberdyne headquarters in summer 2009, he highlighted the innovative aspects of HAL and its ability to "support, expand, and enhance human abilities." He said that he and his colleagues were working at the frontier of a multidisciplinary field that he called Cybernics, of which the HAL exoskeleton was but one expression. Like every other roboticist I met, he led me through a set of PowerPoint slides to introduce his work. He began by describing the intention of Cybernics to "create technologies that join together human and machine." The realization of HAL technology, he stressed, depended on an interdisciplinary understanding of human physiology, mechanical engineering, robotics, and computer science.[6]

As examples of the kinds of human–machine fusion that could result, he showed me prototypes of medical devices in development at Cyberdyne, including experimental pacemakers and wearable heart and blood monitors. When he moved to the HAL exoskeleton, he emphasized its potential to help people with incurable disabilities walk while wearing the suit. He played short video clips of three individuals walking while wearing the suit: one with a spinal cord injury; one with muscular dystrophy; and one with a history of polio. The patient had been stricken with polio as a child and had not walked in decades. The video showed him being connected to the HAL lower-body suit, slowly rising from a wheelchair and walking gingerly while gripping onto horizontal support bars. He walked for several steps and then the video stopped. Prof. Sankai shared with me the man's deeply moving emotional reaction to this experience. The presentation was impressive but it surprised me as well. I had arranged an interview with him because I was interested in how his technology would help older adults, but the presentation did not include images or videos of elderly individuals walking while wearing the suit. The unstated assumption was that frail older adults would benefit from wearing the suit in the same way as persons with walking disabilities. When he did mention the care of older adults, the discussion turned to how wearing HAL might help prevent injuries to nurses as they perform the physically demanding work of caring for others. There was no suggestion that older adults, or people with disabilities for that matter, would wear the suit so that they could learn to walk better without it. This would change not long after we spoke.

Loop Two: Feedback Therapy

In late 2010, officials from the German state of North Rhine–Westphalia invited Dr. Thomas Schildhauer, a surgeon and specialist in the treatment of spinal cord injuries, to attend a presentation on HAL technology by Prof. Sankai. The presentation focused on the contribution HAL could make in caring for a growing elderly population. This was presumably a topic of interest for a German audience—the country has one of the highest per capita populations of seniors in Europe (World Bank 2023). But in an interview with me in 2017, Dr. Schildhauer recalled that most of the assembled civil servants and business leaders were skeptical. Dr. Schildhauer, however, "saw the great potential of [HAL]. Seeing a demonstration for the first time, it occurred to me that this would be a perfect thing for our spinal cord injury patients." Prof. Sankai learned of Dr. Schildhauer's enthusiasm, and invited him to present at a conference in Tokyo in March 2011, just a few days before a devasting earthquake shook Japan. In his presentation, Dr. Schildhauer explained his interest in trialing HAL in the treatment of walking disabilities and also outlined how such care could be financed by BG (Statutory Accident Insurance, discussed later in this chapter). Medical researchers from Sweden and Japan were also present for the doctor's presentation. Conversations among them led to the formation of three national research teams to investigate the utility of HAL in treating walking disabilities: Schildhauer's group in Germany would test its suitability for patients with spinal cord injuries; a team at the Karolinska Institute in Sweden would do the same for stroke patients; and another in Japan would explore applications for patients living with neuromuscular disease.

The launching of three concurrent research projects signaled an important turning point in the development of HAL technology, one that demonstrates again the loose connection between discourses on the aging society and the development of Japanese care robotics. The HAL suit would no longer be developed, if it ever was, primarily around the needs of aging bodies. Instead, development would proceed in response to the needs of bodies impaired by injury or disease. Schildhauer had presented Sankai with this new direction as well as a viable financial path forward (BG insurance). The path was not yet certain but it provided the Japanese inventor, and soon patients, therapists, doctors, businessmen, and engineers, with a new capacity to aspire.

Clinical trials began in Germany in 2012. The team received preliminary approval to test the device with a small sample of carefully supervised patients. This first required a minor redesign of the HAL exoskeleton to fit the relatively larger bodies of Germans. Production disruptions caused by the lingering effects of the March 2011 triple disasters in Japan delayed the start of the trials, but by 2013 they had returned results that demonstrated the safety of the device sufficiently enough that it earned a CE mark. (A "CE" mark indicates that a product is safe for use and can be sold within the EU. Unlike approval by the FDA, it does not certify efficacy.) A more robust clinical trial commenced following receipt of the CE mark. Those trials were, according to Schildhauer, "very, very promising."

Over the course of these and future trials, the German team would discover that repeated sessions of walking with HAL increased the mobility of some patients with partial spinal cord injuries even when they were not wearing the robot suit. The reasons why are not precisely understood, but clinical data suggests that they result from changes in the brain. Even more striking, the mechanism that is believed to bring about these changes is the same as that by which HAL senses and responds: feedback. One member of the team described the process as follows.

> Whenever you have a spinal cord injury where some signals are going into your lower limbs, then the HAL system can recognize these signals, although you might not be strong enough to move your muscles. If they can't move your muscles, then you are wheelchair-bound. But these signals can be sensed, then trigger a motor in the HAL system, and you can walk. Then your brain learns that whenever it's sending signals to implement a motion or movement, then it gets a reaction. *And that's a*

feedback system . . . Whenever you have a circle, *a closed loop,* with a short enough lag time, then your brain learns again to accept that. If the lag is too long, then the learning is not as good. The loop needs to be closed and fast. Then you get interconnections in your brain again. You may get interconnections above and below the level of the spinal cord injury, and with training your muscle is getting stronger again. Nerve endings in the muscle are sprouting . . . These effects are the reason why patients benefit from HAL training. (my emphasis)

Although Dr. Schildhauer and his colleagues work primarily with spinal cord injury patients, what the doctor describes above is akin to what Japanese researchers testing HAL with stroke patients describe as "interactive biofeedback" (Morishita and Inoue 2016) and "cybernic neurorehabilitation" (Nakajima 2016). These terms each reflect clinical findings that feedback from conscious recognition of movement while wearing the HAL suit, in addition to the unconscious loops of feedback between brain, body, and machine, is a basis of healing.

In interviews with me, German medical researchers were careful to describe their experiments in terms of symptoms, interventions, and results, without speculating on exactly what in the brain and body responds to feedback. The leading hypothesis, however, is that an adaptive capacity of the brain—"neuroplasticity"—is responsible for changes in function. As one doctor told me, "We can show in fMRI [functional magnetic resonance imaging] scans that there is a recurrence to normal neuroplasticity in the brain." By this he means a phenomenon that often accompanies injuries causing paralysis in the limbs where regions of the brain that were previously responsible for controlling those limbs get taken over ("colonized" in medical parlance) by other parts of the body. After multiple sessions walking with HAL, those colonized areas of the brain appear to return to their former functionality, which, in turn, correlates with greater functionality in the paralyzed limb(s).

The effectiveness of therapy with HAL is measured by changes in physical *function* that begin in the brain, rather than on the repair of spinal cord lesions that are the proximate cause of paralysis. Changes in the plastic brain enhance the functionality of the injured body *without actually healing the body itself.* Feedback between HAL and the human body, that is, does not just establish a closed loop that maintains a steady state of operation. The mobility afforded by the HAL–human assemblage feeds back, through repetition, toward the incremental recovery of physical function. This is care as iteration: it aspires to incremental advancements in physical function through training, not the recovery of physical integrity through surgery. Care as iteration fuels the aspirations of patients. It motivates doctors as well. Those whom I met made sure to emphasize that their conclusions so far were tentative.[7] They stressed the need for more studies, more participants, and more data in order to identify other patients who might benefit from training with HAL and to understand better the physiological mechanisms at work. Their desire to know more contributes to the atmosphere of aspiration that pervades CCR.

Loop Three: Cyberdyne Care Robotics

The promising results of clinical trials with HAL led administrators at Bergmannsheil Hospital to help fund the establishment of Cyberdyne Care Robotics in 2013. The facility is located in Bochum, a small city on the northern bank of the Ruhr River between larger Dortmund to the east and Duisburg-Essen to the west. The population of the Ruhr Valley region surged in the nineteenth century when laborers arrived to mine its rich coal deposits for the nation's industrializing economy. Work in the mines was lucrative but dangerous, and accidents occurred often. In 1890, Bergmannsheil (lit. "miner's health") Hospital opened to provide specialty care for mining injuries. Today, the hospital maintains a reputation in the treatment of traumatic injury and is one of thirteen hospitals administered by the German Statutory Accident Insurance Agency (*Berufsgenossenschaftiches*, abbrv. BG).[8]

CCR sits just across a narrow street from the Bergsmannsheil Hospital. It is housed, appropriately enough, in a renovated coal-storage building. Inside, no trace of the building's heritage in industry remains. Sunlight streams in from tall windows and reflects up from light-colored tiles onto bright white walls. A row of in-floor treadmills set in front of floor-to-ceiling mirrors fills one side of the expansive room. Young trainers float about dressed casually in black tops, white pants, and sneakers. The sleek interior, like that of HAL Fit in Japan, is hard to distinguish from an ordinary fitness club. Support harnesses hanging over treadmills and a row of treatment tables, however, suggest that it is not a typical gym. So do the HAL exoskeletons propped up on stands in an adjoining room, their shiny white plastic shells mirroring the surfaces surrounding them. The very obverse of sooty black, CCR presents a blank canvas on which to imagine a future beyond the traumas inscribed on the body by the past.

The building housing CCR is split administratively into two parts. One is occupied by the headquarters of Cyberdyne Care Robotics; the other by the Center for Neurorobotic Movement Training (*Zentrum für neurorobotales Bewegungstraining*, or ZNB). CCR is a for-profit subsidiary of HAL's manufacturer in Japan, Cyberdyne, Inc. It is a central node in the distribution of Cyberdyne technologies throughout Europe. ZNB is a nonprofit entity that treats patients with the HAL suit after they have completed conventional rehabilitative therapy. ZNB is furthered subdivided into an activity room and an evaluation room. In practice, there is regular movement of patients, staff, and even HAL technology across ZNB and CCR. Clinicians flow between the site and Bergmannsheil Hospital to consult with patients and oversee studies. For sake of brevity, I refer collectively to the facility as CCR, but the ways in which it works to provide care, support knowledge, and spur innovation are made clearer by considering the kinds of activities that take place within its internal divisions.

Patients are made aware of the relationship between CCR and clinical research as soon as they enter the evaluation room of ZNB to start training with HAL. In the middle of the room, there is a stretch of red test track that extends ten meters long by one meter wide. To the left of the track is a waiting area for patient helpers and a small changing area with four stretchers. On the wall to the right of the track, leaning against the wall next to two tripods, are crutches and other walking aids. Above them are framed copies of studies with the HAL suit conducted by doctors at Bergmannsheil, one of which was completed just two weeks before I visited for the second time in July 2017.[9]

In the evaluation room, patients undergo pre-training and post-training tests of physical function. These tests provide quantitative baselines that make it possible to measure the effect of training with HAL. At their initial visit, if they can handle the strain, patients perform a six-minute walking test, which measures walking ability and aerobic capacity. They next perform a Timed Up and Go (TUG) test that records how long it takes for a patient to move from sitting in a chair to standing up and then walking three meters, turning around, and sitting back down in the same chair. This is followed by a standard American Spinal Injury Association (ASIA) assessment of sensory and motor function. Patients repeat these three tests at the conclusion of their final training session with HAL. On regular visits, patients also walk

along the red track before and after sessions with HAL. The degree of assistance they need is scored on a standard Walking Index for Spinal Cord
Injury II (WISC II) scale. A WISC II score is assessed again after they
complete training with HAL for the day.

This battery of tests is required for insurance purposes for all patients, even
for therapies that do not use a HAL suit. At CCR, though, these tests also
standardize individual differences of ability in a way that makes patients comparable in clinical studies. They are recorded on video and saved for individual
consultations as well as research and marketing. On my first visit to CCR, I
was shown several promotional videos about the effectiveness of the HAL
suit that used footage from these recordings. In these videos, patients are presented only by their diagnostic criteria: *Male, 35 years old, Th12/C1 fracture,
complete paraplegic, sub Th12 ASIA A, 3 mos. with HAL, 10m walk test from
72 seconds in 31 steps with assistance to 27 seconds in 20 steps using walker, plus
speed increase of 4km/h to 2.8 km/h.* The same summary data appears in the
reports and presentations of clinical studies with the HAL suit. Reducing patients to standard metrics not only preserves privacy but also makes test results
meaningful for a larger scientific community (and insurers). De-individualizing
the effects of care transforms it into clinical research data that circulates well
beyond the walls of CCR. The process echoes the conversion of care into data
by the Robot Therapy Group in Japan. At CCR, these data become the basis
for future experimental trials and clinical applications of HAL.

For a patient, however, the results of walking tests are far less meaningful
than what happens in the activity room. After walking tests are completed,
therapists attach electrodes on a patient's hips and knees and then wheel
them up a ramp to the activity room. The patient is then strapped into one
of the body-support harnesses hanging over the treadmills. Soon after, the
HAL suit is placed on the patient. Mechanical adjustments are made on the
fly, tightening and loosening as needed. At last, therapists connect electrodes
to the "robot." This establishes a direct connection between the body of the
patient and the exoskeleton, one intended to create a closed loop of feedback.
HAL is designed to work in harmony with the intentions of the patient but it
first needs to be calibrated to individual strengths and limitations.

During calibration, the attention of the therapists moves away from observing the body of the patient to the LED screen on the control module
attached to the HAL suit. The display mediates the movement of the body at
a double remove, converting into visual form the mediation of movement by

the robot, already rendered as digital data. Hence, in training, movements of the body are quantified as they are in the evaluation room. Yet, here quantification points to the concrete. Body and machine are "tuned" to each other, synchronizing the mass-produced machine with the individual body in an effort, ultimately and paradoxically, to extinguish this very individuality. What results is a body–machine assemblage that moves unlike the body without the machine and unlike the machine without a body. For all intents and purposes, the duality is treated as a unity. HAL *qua* feeling machine should not be felt, supporting its own weight and the movement of the body without calling attention to this intermediation (figure 5.1).

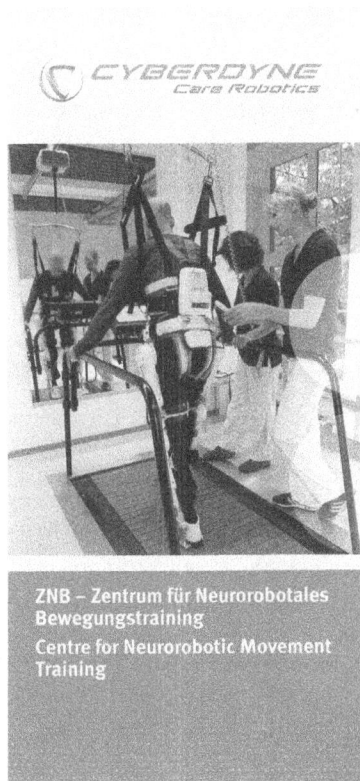

FIGURE 5.1 Training with HAL.   Cover image of a brochure advertising the services of CCR in Germany. The picture shows a patient walking on an in-floor treadmill while attached to a HAL lower-body exoskeleton and supported by a harness. Two therapists stand beside him, with one watching an LED display of HAL's operation on an attached control module. Photo used courtesy of Cyberdyne Care Robotics.

The activity room may be oriented to the concrete needs of the individual patient, but the data it generates also flows out of CCR, not in the service of academic research but in the interest primarily of corporate innovation. HAL suits send digitized training data to servers at Cyberdyne headquarters in Japan, where it is stored, aggregated, and processed. This is ostensibly done for the benefit of patients, who might gain insights from the computational analysis of their training sessions over multiple sessions. Yet therapists at CCR do not have access to this data nor can they see what data is being transmitted. I did not observe references to this information in sessions with HAL, nor did I hear about its use in interviews with staff. Staff members at CCR and at Cyberdyne in Japan, however, told me that training data is of value to engineers who can use it to assess the functional strengths and limitations of HAL technology.[10]

The feedback loops of the HAL–human assemblage at CCR are, in reality, far from closed. Data generated by the assemblage flows out from CCR in the service of clinical research and technological development. The digital connections between HAL suits in Germany and corporate servers in Japan demonstrate the intensification of connections between care sites and corporate sites examined in previous chapters. Loops of feedback that constitute the HAL–human assemblage are transformed almost immediately into spirals of open innovation, making CCR at once a space of care, a site of clinical research, and a platform for technological innovation.

Loops Closed, Loops Broken

For patients I met at CCR, however, it was the achievement of a properly functioning closed loop that made the strongest impression. They described with excitement and elation the first time they felt the HAL–human assemblage operate as it should. A patient named Janet relayed to me her initial impressions.

In the beginning it was hard because we had to find the proper settings. Once we did, then I could walk with this machine quite well. Of course, when you first put HAL on and try walking, you feel that you have this machine on. But after a few steps, you don't feel the weight anymore—it just supports *(unterstützen)* you. It really helps and doesn't bother you. It's quite good. It feels like a part of me, like I don't have to think I just try to walk. And, if the settings are correct, then that's easy to manage.

"It feels like a part of me" was a sentiment I heard often. In an interview, Jenny, the young woman whose training session starts the chapter, expressed her experience in precisely these terms. She described further how sessions with HAL help her recover memories of her former self—a feeling produced, ironically, by a selective forgetting of her body's current state (what she calls "tricking" or "cheating" her brain).

> At first, my steps were a little uncertain. I could feel the weight of the machine. But after a few steps, I felt like before the accident. I felt good and strong and free. I felt more fit—it's not just training for the legs. I felt like I could walk lots of meters and it'd be no problem. The robot [*roboter*—i.e., HAL] helps me train the muscles so much. So, I work with this robotic suit a half hour on and it's, well, the brain works with it, so it's . . . hard to explain, but, yeah, the brain doesn't realize [that I'm attached to a] robot. The brain thinks that I'm walking on my own and . . . so after the first few months I trust my legs more. It's kind of like tricking the brain, cheating the brain. Now it feels like it's a part of me. It's cool!

What Janet and Jenny describe is a kind of reverse uncanny. Rather than feeling anxious when something familiar suddenly seems unfamiliar, the classic uncanny as conceptualized by Freud, tuning HAL led to moments when a body that feels disconnected, that doesn't respond as you remember or you would like, instantly feels like it does—"it feels like a part of me."[11] These feelings of physical integrity, though technologically mediated, draw on images of futuristic cyborgs already present in the imaginations of those who experience them. They recall Prof. Sankai's excitement about achieving the "fusion" of human and machine through HAL technology. But, if these are moments worth remembering, they are set among moments of forgetting in the course of HAL training. Feelings of liberation when the closed loop works occur among frequent episodes of disruption and disconnection when it breaks. Sessions with HAL are marked by instances of failure and correction, of tinkering on the fly to manage exigencies of body and machine. These lend sessions with HAL an air of ad hoc experimentation, extending the atmosphere of experimentation in the evaluation room into training sessions.

Janet's training session is instructive. The day I observe is Janet's first day back at CCR since taking a two-week vacation. Janet is a thirty-two-year-old postdoctoral researcher in an institute of neurology in nearby Dortmund. Around the age of fifteen, she noticed that she occasionally had difficulty walking. Her symptoms progressed, and Janet eventually needed braces and other aids to walk. Doctors could not identify the cause of her walking impairment. They referred her for physical therapy on the assumption that muscle weakness or some other impingement might be at fault. Nothing seemed to help. Then, one day a few years before I met her, she noticed a red band around her waist that looked like a burn. At the hospital, doctors discovered that she had a cavernoma, a benign tumor of the nervous system, lodged in her spinal column that had been bleeding slowly for years. Pressure from this bleeding had been causing her mysterious symptoms. Doctors surgically removed the cavernoma but the operation left her with terrible spasms in her legs, particularly her right one. She sought the advice of neurologists at Bergmannsheil, who told her about HAL training and recommended that she visit CCR. She enrolled in one of their research studies (which helped to defray the considerable cost of the training). Sessions with HAL made a dramatic difference for her.

> [HAL] really helps me, because afterwards I really feel better. The spasm is really reduced and then I'm ready for work (laughs). Since I work in a lab, I need to walk. If I went to work without first training with HAL, I would need a couple of hours just to adjust. After training with HAL, I can immediately start working. It's really cool. I mean I've been doing physical therapy since I was fifteen, but no amount of physical therapy has helped me as much as the last eight weeks working with HAL. It's really the most effective therapy I have ever had. I feel much happier. I mean, what makes me happy is that I can do something now that I couldn't do before, and that . . . that's amazing.

On the day I observe, Janet is placed in the HAL suit and Suzette, her therapist, checks its operation. Is it registering signals from Janet's body appropriately? Something's wrong. Suzette traces the issue to a malfunctioning sensor on one leg. She swaps it out for a new one, and checks signals again. The signals seem weaker than they were on previous visits. Suzette adjusts the sensitivity settings of the machine to compensate. She starts the treadmill at a slow pace.

Janet tries to walk and, in so doing, activates the mechanical support of HAL. She grabs the support bars of the treadmill tightly. Straining to move her legs to keep pace with the speed of the treadmill, she scrutinizes herself in the mirror on the wall in front of her. This form of visual monitoring, therapists tell me, is vital in helping patients improve functional ability. Patients need to see themselves moving their legs as much as their bodies need to sense them moving their legs in a way that is not possible without HAL support. Even as she struggles, a smile remains fixed on Janet's face.

Suzette (S): It looks like the left foot is functioning well today.

Janet (J): Yes . . . but it's hard.

S: Of course, but it's really good. Okay, step forward. Forward! (Turning to me) She's had a lot of leg spasms in the last two days. She'll have a botox injection (which helps decrease their frequency) on Friday.

After a few minutes, Suzette decides to give Janet a break. Janet remains on the treadmill, standing and holding onto the support bars. Another therapist checks her pulse and blood pressure. They chat for a bit.

S: Are you having a good time?

J: It's been two weeks. It's hard starting again.

S: Of course it is. Give it a few more times. It's always this way when restarting.

The short break ends and Suzette starts up the treadmill again.

S: Left is perfect. Try to pick right up higher! Good . . . Forward . . . Forward. Good . . . Forward . . . Keep going! Good! Exactly. Not so loud! [a reference to how hard she is putting her foot down on the treadmill.]. Keep more control on the right side! One more minute. Let's go! Forward . . . Forward . . . Up! High knees! Okay, thirty seconds left. Yes, good. A little farther. Let's go! Okay, and stop. Good!

Suzette stops the treadmill. Janet steps off of the treadmill and sits on a chair. Suzette checks Janet's pulse and blood pressure.

S: How are you doing? Good?

J: I'm warm.

S: That's normal. Where do you feel it when you push your leg forward or bring it back?

J: Both.

S: In the knee or in the hip?

J: Both.

Suzette helps her back on the stationary treadmill and tells Janet to work on her balance. Without touching the machine, Suzette has Janet squat down and up while keeping her back straight. Janet repeats this several times. Sat-isfied, Suzette restarts the treadmill and Janet begins walking again. After a few minutes, Suzette ducks under the bars of the treadmill and puts her open palm out in front of Janet's right foot. She tells Janet to try to touch her hand with her foot—"Kick my hand! Forward! Yes . . . Exactly. Use your stom-ach muscles!" Suzette notices that Janet is still struggling to push her right foot forward enough. She grabs the metal bar between the lower end of the exoskeleton frame and its shoe. She pushes Janet's right leg forward toward full extension. "Forward . . . Use your stomach muscles . . . Good! . . . Right foot . . . Right foot . . . Forward!"

Therapists often physically support patients wearing the HAL suit. They hold the waist frame as patients walk on treadmills, grab the upper-leg frame of the exoskeleton to help patients lift their knees higher, or, like Suzette, push the metal rod between the lower-leg frame to guide one leg forward. In so doing, therapists became part of the assemblage of patient and HAL in a manner more directly tactile than monitoring a digital display. But this does not mean that HAL no longer mediates such interactions between patients and therapists. In these moments, I only observed therapists touching parts of the HAL exoskeleton, not the bodies of patients, as if tacitly confirming that HAL was mediating the therapeutic encounter between them and pa-tients, both digitally and mechanically. By contrast, before and after attach-ing HAL to patients, therapists frequently touch patients both informally (e.g., patting them on the shoulders or back for encouragement) and formally (e.g., helping them stretch and loosen up in preparation for training).

Suzette helps Janet move her right leg forward for a few more minutes, until Janet indicates that she needs a bathroom break. Two therapists work together quickly to remove the HAL suit and the support harness. Janet hops off the treadmill and uses crutches to go to the bathroom. While she's there, one of the therapists turns to me: "She's regressed after her two-week break. Both in her walking and also in her training. She can't sense ahead of time when she needs to go to the bathroom. She has to go immediately, like when it's an emergency."

Patients with spinal cord injuries leading to paralysis of the lower limbs often become incontinent. But therapists and doctors both told me that pa-tients mention improvements in peripheral organ function as their walking ability increases. Along with strengthening nerve connections between the brain and muscles in the lower extremities, they speculate, HAL training even seems to enhance signal pathways between the brain and other organs below the point of injury. Janet's regression indicates, however, that these enhancements are not necessarily permanent. One can lose them, which heightens the imperative to continue regular training in order to maintain physical function.

Janet returns from the bathroom. Suzette and another therapist take about ten minutes to put the harness and HAL back on Janet. They help Janet get back up on the treadmill, and Suzette restarts the treadmill at a slow speed. She notices that something is still not right. She stops the treadmill, grabs a screwdriver, and adjusts the fit of the HAL suit on her left side. Janet has a tendency to swing her left foot in a bit. By modifying how the HAL suit fits, Suzette tries to straighten out the arc of her left leg.

Suzette restarts the treadmill and stays behind Janet, as if she is watching her walk. But she doesn't look at Janet. Instead, head hanging down, she watches animated representations of Janet's body on the LED display. These show her transition through the various phases of walking programmed into the HAL machine. Outlines of her left foot and right foot glow red as the foot-pressure sensor registers shifts in body weight.

S: Scrunch those abs! Keep your back straight! Keep it strong! That good? Is that better?

J: Maybe . . .

Suzette encourages Janet to focus on her walking. Like other patients, many of whom are weaker than she, Janet sometimes grips the support bars too tightly in an attempt to use her upper-body strength to whip her legs forward instead of using her leg muscles. Patients who normally use wheelchairs or other walking aids to move around tend not to "trust" their legs, even when they are on a treadmill and are supported by the combination of harness and HAL. They compensate by forcing their upper bodies to do the work, just as they must do when they are not on the treadmill. Therapists exhort their patients to "trust their bodies" and to "walk with their legs, not with their arms." Without "trusting" one's legs and trying to walk, patients not only fail to see an increase in mobility but HAL itself will not function correctly: HAL cannot do anything without a body; it is activated only by the intended movements of a patient aspiring for yet more mobility.

As if on cue, a loud buzz and rattle starts to emanate from Janet's right foot. Her expression, which appeared frozen in a permanent smile, suddenly constricts in strain and frustration. Looking down, I see her right foot jerk-ing rapidly back and forth. Her leg has gone into spasm. Suzette stops the treadmill and ducks under the handrail to grab the metal bar near the HAL robot's shoe. She tells Janet to try to relax. Another therapist steps up and taps controls on the machine's console to reduce the amount of support it pro-vides. Janet's leg gradually stops lurching and the noise of vibration recedes. "Okay, try to walk again . . ." Suzette moves back behind Janet and restarts the treadmill, gradually dialing up supplemental support from HAL.

Spasm, a condition that is common in people with spinal cord injuries, reveals much about the principles of HAL's operation. The functionality of HAL is premised on intentional control by the wearer. Even if control signals (i.e., nerve impulses) are weak, its makers claim, HAL can sense and amplify them to make movement possible. In theory, HAL works by sensing the cir-culation of nerve signals between limb and machine. This theory assumes a smooth flow of nerve signals (information) within the body (a closed loop), from brain (control unit) to limb (actuator). The body in spasm disrupts this system. When part of the body is in spasm, flexion and extension of mus-cles are triggered at the same time. HAL's voluntary control system cannot separate signal from noise, or, more appropriate to this case, disentangle an excess of signals pointing in contradictory directions, leading to malfunction. The only way to resolve the malfunction entirely is to decrease the amount of support HAL provides or to interrupt the closed loop by separating person from machine. HAL "sees" the body as a closed system, like a circuit board. But bodies are not circuit boards. Spasm that causes mechanical malfunc-tion reveals how assemblages of bodies and brains (and machines connected to them) exist in perpetual tension, unities always on the verge of breaking down.

If spasm throws into question the analogies of human and machine that guide HAL's operation, neuropathic pain does the same for the effect of training with the suit. Neuropathic pain is common in patients with spinal cord injuries. It is akin to the "phantom pain" that amputees often feel in limbs that have been amputated. People with injuries to the spinal cord can experience chronic, neuropathic pain in parts of their body where they oth-erwise have little to no sensation. Such pain unsettles beliefs about the unity of body and mind—how is it possible to feel something in a part of the body that no longer works or is not even there?

Over the course of training with HAL, patients often report that the intensity of neuropathic pain diminishes. Doctors and therapists suggest that strengthening signal flow between brain and limb in HAL training helps resolve adjacent neuropathic pain. They view it as a salutary but unpredictable side effect, one that they proudly mention in research reports and presentations (see Cruciger et al. 2016). Yet the presence of neuropathic pain, like spasm, undermines a view of the body as nothing more than an organic network of sensors and actuators connected to a control unit. A sensor network that does not exist cannot send signals or malfunction, but a phantom limb can register phantom pain. If spasm disrupts the operation of HAL *because* it senses intention too precisely and fails to "read" its contradictions, no amount of engineering will make HAL capable of intentionally targeting phantom pain that it can never sense.

Janet is now walking again. Suzette returns her gaze to the LED display. After a few minutes, she brings the console around the side of the treadmill so Janet can see it. Suzette points out that Janet should move her foot in a rocking motion, from heel to toe. Patients have a tendency to put their feet down flat, smacking them against the surface of the treadmill, as Janet is doing now, instead of rocking heel to toe.

S: Focus on going heel-toe on your left foot. Bigger steps on the right. (shouting) High knee! Forward!

Like watching one's movement in a mirror, therapists believe that monitoring a real-time, virtual representation of walking—split-second changes in the amount of mechanical support, fluctuations in the strength of nerve signals, shifts in pressure on the soles of one's feet—can strengthen the feedback effect of the suit, providing greater recognition *in the moment* of what it feels like to walk. Some therapists even wished that the activity room had big LED screens mounted beside the wall mirrors, as some HAL Fit sites do in Japan (see chapter 2). At the same time, once patients demonstrate some improvement in their ability to walk, therapists often turn them away from the mirror and have them toss or kick balls back-and-forth so that they concentrate less on trying to walk. The intention is to help return the conscious effort to move one's legs to the unconscious process it should be.

Suzette moves back behind Janet and looks down again at the LED display. Seemingly satisfied at what she sees, she places the console back on the waist of the exoskeleton. She grabs a camcorder off of a tripod that is set up nearby and begins recording Janet walking on the treadmill (recording happens in the training room, too). This continues for about five minutes.

> S: Good! Good progress! How are you feeling?
> J: Um . . . I understand the feeling of walking better.
> S: Ok, thirty more seconds and we can end on a good note. [slowing the treadmill down] Okay . . . 5, 4, 3, 2, 1. Stop! Super . . . That was a good round. For you, too?
> J: Yeah.
> S: How do you feel after walking?
> J: Out of breath.

Suzette detaches HAL from Janet but has her stay harnessed on the treadmill. Suzette starts the treadmill once again and has Janet try to walk without HAL's support. Suzette leans down and holds the back of Janet's leg, pushing her right foot forward as she tries to take a step. Janet works hard to keep up, but looks stronger than she did when she initially started the session. Still, HAL is not far from their minds. Joking, Suzette lightly taps Janet's right hip and says, "Activate it! Activate it!"

After a few more minutes, it's time to stop. Suzette helps Janet out of the harness and has her sit back in a chair. Janet appears relieved to be off the treadmill and thrilled about her workout. After a brief rest, she takes a pair of crutches under her arms and walks back to the evaluation room to perform her walking tests. The intensely subjective experience of training, all the attention given to the experience of the patients during training—How are you? Do you need a break? Is that too hard?—now shifts to an objective remove.

Plastic Minds, Plastic Futures

For patients, the results of ten-meter walking tests or TUG tests are rarely meaningful. Patient aspirations are grounded in concrete experiences in everyday life. After she finishes cooling down, I talk with Janet about what she hopes to achieve by training with HAL. "Well, at first, I *wanted* to walk without crutches! But now, sometimes, I can walk without them . . . Like if I'm in a small room, I can grab something from a cupboard and take it to a table, or something like that. I can manage that now. But I think I need more training to walk without them! (laughs)." I follow up, "Do you think another month (until training ends) will be enough time? "I hope so," she says with a laugh, "but probably not!"

Janet's sentiments are shared by others whom I meet. Jenny, whose spinal cord was partially severed in a horse-riding accident, tells me about the transformation that she experienced after training with HAL for several months:

> After training in the beginning, it felt good to walk here but I was a bit scared to use crutches at home. But now I use crutches more often, or stand up to take a glass from a high shelf. I stand up to pick something up, or to stand up to see something, because, when I sit the whole day, I just look at the hallway (laughs). If I'm in a room with a chair or something I can hold onto, then I can take a few steps with my hand here or there, or stand for five minutes or so. The other day we were at a festival and I stood up to see the band . . .
>
> There was a moment over Christmas where my parents and I realized how much progress I'd made after just a couple of months. I was flying on a plane and needed to go to the bathroom. I was able to stand up and walk all the way to the bathroom, supporting myself on the backs of seats. It was a special moment. My parents and I saw that I could apply this therapy to different things, not just walking ten meters like I do here. So, everyday life is more normal again.
>
> With more training, my goal is to manage the two or three steps it takes to get into a house. Like, I feel bad when I come to a house and can't manage to walk in . . . and, of course, I want to improve the quality of my walking. My dream is to have a normal day without the wheelchair. Like, to get up from the couch to go get coffee . . . I know I can't walk an hour with the dog outside. That's unrealistic. But in small ways, in the everyday, yeah, I don't want to have to use the wheelchair.

Two years before I met Ralph, he was in a motorcycle accident. The front tire of his motorcycle hit the rear tire of another motorcyclist at a traffic stop. The motorcycle flipped over, catapulting him over the handlebars and then crashing down on him. The accident left him with fractured second and third thoracic vertebrae in addition to partial paralysis of his lower limbs, what a staff member at CCR called "a classic spinal cord injury." His injuries were so severe that the hospital to which he was first admitted transferred him to specialists at Bergmannsheil, where he had surgery and lay in a coma for ten weeks. After five months of conventional rehabilitation, a doctor encouraged him to try HAL training, but his leg muscles were still too weak for him to handle walking in the HAL suit. He completed additional therapy and was now strong enough to walk for a few minutes with the suit on.

Watching him train with HAL, it was apparent that he still had much difficulty walking. "Without HAL I cannot move at all, so everything on the treadmill is premeditated. I have to think about every step," he told me. He took frequent breaks. His therapists would help him off the treadmill, seat him in a chair, and then hand him a bottle of Coke to sip. He hoped that someday he might be able "to maybe walk a few meters again." But ultimately, and much like Janet and Jenny, he had a very concrete goal in mind. "My goal is," he continued, "to ride in my wheelchair to my car, bring it inside, get in the driver's seat, and drive a car." If this didn't happen by the end of his training with HAL, he told me further, "then I'll wait a little longer. I'll keep on. Steady, steady. Easy, easy."

Like Jenny and Janet, Ralph does not aim for a return to the "normal." A return to the way things once were, they all realize, is impossible. Instead, they approach improvement incrementally, toward "a more normal day." A few steps to the house. Up from the couch to get coffee. Navigating an aisle to get to the airplane bathroom by herself. Driving a car. Carving more time during the day for independent mobility. Each movement forward is a step toward another. The future is set iteratively, a terminus perpetually deferred.

———————

For those patients with spinal cord injury, the trauma of "the accident" is a clear temporal dividing line between a past of independent mobility and a present of diminished independence and mobility. For individuals I met whose mobility had been impaired by an apparent neuromuscular disorder, the temporal dividing line is not so clear. Difficulties with walking emerge much more gradually. These individuals nevertheless express similar sentiments about the point of their training. Gunther, who at age sixty-two was one of the oldest people I met at CCR, began experiencing difficulties with balance and coordination at the age of thirty. He saw a number of doctors in the years following and, while some speculated that he might have a new kind of disease, none felt confident diagnosing him. Gunther's symptoms progressed over the years, so much so that he found he had difficulty controlling his walking. He would collapse suddenly or fall over if he leaned down to pick something up. Even standing straight became difficult for him. A doctor at Bergmannsheil referred him to CCR where he was enrolled in a research study (which paid for his training sessions). When I met him, he had just completed eight weeks of training at ZNB. He found that he had gotten closer to the goal of controlling his physical movements.

> When I walk now by myself, I can do so more consciously. Previously, I could only go a few meters before feeling like I might fall and I had little strength in my legs and arms. Now, I can move more intentionally, with more control. When I train with HAL, I feel like I am accomplishing something athletic. I feel that I have more strength, and that I move better. I am not kept awake by pain as much as I was before. My digestion is even better!

Heinrich's symptoms, though seemingly neuromuscular, emerged much more suddenly than Gunther's. An eighty-four-year-old retired architect, Heinrich liked to hike in the mountains where the clean air and lack of allergens moderated his asthma symptoms. On a trip to the Austrian Alps in 2003, he awoke one morning without any energy. He made it out of bed but soon found that he couldn't take more than a few steps, even with a cane. He remained in the hotel convalescing for an additional two weeks. Then began, he told me, "the tragedy of the neurologists." He met with many specialists at many different hospitals. They ruled out Parkinson's disease but nobody could identify a cause. One day he happened to see an article in a German newspaper on a prototype walking aid from Honda in Japan. He went so far as to contact the company to see if their device might help him. "They sent me some papers filled with drawings of people walking around outside with leg exoskeletons." He added, dejectedly, "They told me to wait five years. And, well, it's been more than five years!" Heinrich was put on an opioid-based medication for Parkinson's patients to help him manage his symptoms. Though helpful, he still worried about falling. Just the week before I met him, he fell on the sidewalk, injuring his hip and badly bruising his hand. "My father got to seventy-nine in perfect health. And then in eight days he was dead. But not me. I've had to deal with this shit for years!" he said, exasperated.

While the exact cause of Heinrich's walking impairments remains elusive, he was eventually referred to CCR. When I met him in 2017, Heinrich visited CCR at least once a week. He was beloved by staff, who enjoyed listening to him talk about his many travels and his life in wartime Germany. Heinrich talked to me about the feeling he gets when he works with HAL—"It is a part of me." Just being able to move with the suit gives him exercise and conditioning that he cannot obtain elsewhere. After training, he finds that he can stand up straighter than usual, albeit not for long. He can walk farther and more confidently than at the start of training. This is evident in the differences between his pre- and post-training ten-meter tests: "from thirty steps to twenty steps, with much longer steps," his therapist told me.

Unlike patients with traumatic injuries, Heinrich has been dealing for years with symptoms from an undiagnosed illness but retains an enviable level of independence. He can still drive and get around on his own with a walker or cane. Unlike patients with spinal cord injuries who aspire to increased functionality, Heinrich is motivated by the fear of *losing* mobility, especially since the absence of a confident diagnosis of his condition makes a "cure" unlikely. While he does not believe that a return to his "normal" self is likely, it remains for him something of an ultimate dream. Heinrich strives for more concrete outcomes. He wants to be able to accept more of the many invitations he and his wife receive from friends to socialize. When socializing, he wants to stand up and talk with them eye to eye. "When I meet everybody, I first have to sit down in a chair. All the conversation goes on above me. Later, my wife tells me what everyone said." Heinrich's concrete goals echo those of another man with a spinal cord injury who came to train with HAL at CCR. His goal was simply to be able to stand up at the bar for a few minutes and talk with his friends face to face. For this man and for Heinrich, the complete restoration of mobility remains out of reach, but working with HAL fosters in both of them the capacity to aspire to goals that were deemed achievable.

Conversations with patients at CCR demonstrated to me just how much training in the activity room is motivated by concrete, incremental goals for improved mobility. In my fieldwork, I only encountered one person who told me that he wished to "walk like before the accident." Matthias was an athletic younger man in his thirties with a wife and daughter. A few months before he came to CCR, he was involved in a three-car pileup while driving to work, which left him with partial paralysis of the lower limbs. When I asked what he hoped to achieve by training with HAL, he raised an eyebrow, chuckled, and said, "I'd like to walk like I did before." The self-effacing laugh was meant for me and the staff person next to me. He wanted us to know that he understood how unrealistic this hope was. He quickly added a more specific list of goals he thought was more realistic. "No, I'd like to be able to walk without a walker, to go shopping with my wife and daughter, maybe walk a little bit farther."

Therapists I met told me that Matthias's desire for a recovery of past mobility is not uncommon among new patients. Patients often come to CCR soon after exhausting therapeutic options elsewhere or not long after a traumatic accident, often under the misapprehension that HAL will be able to fix their impairment and return them to normal function. Therapists told me about how they carefully work to help patients ratchet down their expectations. This often requires several visits as patients gradually realize the time it takes to tune HAL correctly. After observing how they perform in initial training sessions, therapists work with patients to devise more realistic goals for their months of training at CCR.

The concrete goals I heard expressed in my conversations with patients at CCR are the product of negotiations between therapists and patients over time. This analog feedback mirrors the digital feedback loops underlying the operation of the HAL suit. Together they activate the bodies of patients and motivate their will to engage with the robot suit in the first place. They enhance the capacity of patients to aspire toward a future of incrementally more mobility, one whose horizon advances outward to match and then exceed the functional capacity of bodies training with HAL.

Branding Loops, Bureaucratic Hoops

At CCR, it is understood that this vision of the future-as-plastic does not apply just to brains and bodies. Therapists and patients are aware that the HAL suits that they use every day are in a process of becoming otherwise. They see themselves as engaging with HAL at one moment along a continuum of the machine's development, which provides them something in the present and promises something greater in the future. As the capabilities of the technology expand, so does their capacity to aspire. Patients want a version of the suit that they can wear outside or at home, free from the constraints of safety harnesses. Therapists want large LED screens that mirror the displays on their control consoles so patients can observe subtle shifts in movement and response, heightening the feedback effect of training. They want shoes that are not stiff but allow the ankle to flex, which would make it even easier for patients to relearn walking. Doctors and even some patients dream of a day when the technology is so thin and light it could be worn like clothing. Heinrich put it best: "Well, I think the whole thing [HAL] is just fantastic. I believe that it has a bright future . . . past my own existence . . . into the next generation," he told me. "Naturally, of course, technology is always invented when one is too old."

Managers at CCR, too, look forward to a future with HAL, but they think less about its technical iteration than its potential application to new diseases, new classes of patients, and new insurance markets. One of the first people I met on my initial visit to CCR in 2015 was Mr. Buch, then managing director of the organization. Mr. Buch looked every part the executive. A tall, portly man in his fifties, he dressed like a corporate hipster in his twenties: navy-blue blazer, crisp white oxford shirt with collar open to the chest, skinny-fit blue jeans, and polished black shoes. When I asked how he came to be involved in CCR, I expected to hear him recall a long history in the fields of healthcare or technology. Instead, he told me about his many years working in the mining insurance industry as an executive. This experience led him to an executive position at a hospital affiliated with the BG system. In 2010, the insurance system that covers mining merged with six other systems to form the BG RCI (Statutory Accident Insurance System for the Raw Materials and Chemical Industry, *Berufsgenossenschaft Rohstoffe und Chemische Industrie*). Mr. Buch left a position at the hospital to work at BG RCI headquarters, housed in a building adjacent to CCR, until plans for CCR started to develop.

His familiarity with hospital administration and the BG insurance system were attractive to his future German and Japanese colleagues. As he put it to me, "It's not easy to join the Statutory *Health* Insurance System." Statutory *Health* Insurance *(Gesetzliche Krankenkasse)* is, of course, distinct from Statutory Accident Insurance. The latter is similar in principle to workmen's compensation insurance in the United States (in fact, the US program is based on the German model, which was first in the world): employers pay into a common insurance fund; employees who are injured on the job—or on the way to or from work—can qualify for benefits; and employees receive benefits not just until they are "healthy" but up to the time that they are able to return to work. Accident insurance permits reimbursement for a greater range of therapies than health insurance, as long as it is conducted under the supervision of a physician, and HAL training is one of the therapies eligible for reimbursement. Many spinal cord injuries result from accidents on the job, and, Mr. Buch told me, "Paraplegics are a big problem for the BG system.

They have a great need for care that lasts a long time—wheelchairs, walkers, care homes, nurses, and so on." Ableist as it is, his comment suggests that the expense of caring for paraplegics with existing technology is the main reason why the insurance system reimburses training with HAL. If most or all patients who undergo HAL training require less assistance in the long term, the cost of a three-month round of HAL training makes financial sense. And not only does accident insurance ease the financial burdens of care on patients and the state, it also provides CCR with a dependable source of revenue from the operation of HAL suits.

While dependable, it is also minimal. Mr. Buch and the management of CCR want HAL training to be covered by the health insurance system in addition to accident insurance. Their primary objective is a listing of HAL therapy on what they call "the catalog." This "service catalog for health insurance" *(Leistungskatalog der Krankenkasse)* is an inventory of all services and medications that are reimbursable under the German statutory health insurance system. In addition to statutory accident and health insurance, Germany also has approximately one hundred private insurers. While some of these companies covered therapy with HAL at the time of my conversation with Mr. Buch, there was no mandate to do so. A listing in the service catalog would mean that all public and private insurers would have to cover the service.

Everything listed in the catalog must first be approved by an entity called the Federal Joint Committee *(Gemeinsamer Bundeausschuss)*. The process of getting approval is complicated and time-consuming, which is why Mr. Buch's knowledge of the bureaucracy of German statutory insurance had such value. Mr. Buch laid out the organization's strategy for me.

> First, you go to them and then you say, "We have this new treatment. It's called the HAL system." Then, you say, "We've done clinical trials with the system. The results have been this and this, and it's good for patients." Next, you have to show how it will affect patients in hospitals, rehabilitation facilities, or private clinics. Then, you negotiate fees for the service at hospitals, rehabilitation facilities, or private clinics.

For Mr. Buch and executives at CCR, the connection of their company to doctors at a research hospital were highly advantageous. They could quickly conceive clinical applications of the suit, enroll appropriate patients in research studies, and apply the results toward further study or the basis of an

application to the Federal Joint Committee. Research studies at CCR, therefore, have value beyond furthering medical understanding alone. Detailed
biomedical definitions of patient injuries and symptoms do more than just
standardize individual bodies for purposes of scientific comparison. Medical
research helps identify new medical applications of HAL technology. New,
approved clinical applications mean new groups of patients; new groups of
patients mean a bigger market for HAL and bigger profits for CCR and Cyberdyne in Japan.

   In their strategy for approaching the Federal Joint Committee, the
German staff at CCR deviate from the preferred approach of their Japanese
colleagues at Cyberdyne. Their Japanese partners, one manager at CCR told
me, like to highlight the robotic nature of the suit "because it is Dr. Sankai's
baby. *His* robot." While Japanese executives like to stress the cutting-edge
technologies underlying the HAL suit, German managers believe that over-
emphasizing technological uniqueness complicates a prospective application
to the Federal Joint Committee. Doing so would require them to differentiate
HAL from all other lower-body exoskeletons on the market. At the time of
my visit in 2015, these included powered lower-body exoskeletons made by
companies like EksoBionics and ReWalk Robotics. These exoskeletons es-
sentially force the legs to move in a certain way based on the position of hips
and knees. The HAL robot includes this functionality as well (e.g., cybernic
autonomous control), but it also interfaces directly with the nerve signals in
the body in a way that those machines do not. CCR managers also worry that
German officials and the public might harbor some prejudice toward a *robotic*
medical device. They intentionally avoid calling activities at CCR "HAL
therapy" or "robot therapy," despite the fact that I often heard therapists
speak about patients "training with the robot." Careful use of terminology is
especially critical given the names connected with the technology itself. One
manager expressed to me her incredulity when she learned that the device
she has to market to health professionals not only shares the name of a killer
AI from film but is also manufactured by a company associated with the
Terminator.

   Managers at CCR instead chose to emphasize the type of therapy that
HAL's control mechanism affords. They considered adopting the existing
term "biofeedback," which has been in use for decades. They determined that
it is not only too vague but also fundamentally refers to a different process
whereby bodies return to homeostasis from a state of excitation (i.e., from

anxious to relaxed). Ultimately, the managers settled on terminology of their own, "neuromuscular feedback therapy." The neologism highlights the novelty of working with HAL. It also expresses the importance of operational/ therapeutic feedback as well as the brain–body connection that they believe to be distinctive. Strategically, it also permits them to avoid technological comparisons with other exoskeletons.

Together with executives at Cyberdyne, CCR managers devised a path toward securing broad insurance coverage for the newly dubbed neuromuscular feedback therapy, beginning with the expansion of coverage for patients with paraplegia unrelated to work injuries. "They are a small insurance class," Mr. Buch told me. "The effect of HAL for this class of patients is well established. It is very likely that the [health] insurance agency will approve insurance for it." Following this, they aim to expand the classes of patients that can receive coverage incrementally: moving from stroke patients with hemiplegia to patients with other kinds of traumatic brain injuries, then onto patients with chronic and degenerative neuromuscular disease (e.g., muscular dystrophy). Staff at CCR feel confident that coverage for this last group will be quickly forthcoming since any medical intervention that halts the progression of debilitating disease must by law be approved for insurance coverage in Germany.

There is classic business logic at work here. The managers of CCR want to "grow the market" of patients so that they can increase their potential profits. But there is also the presence of the kind of iterative thinking that underlies the perspectives of therapists, patients, and technologists involved with CCR. Expanding the classes of patients that can be treated with HAL must begin with clinical trials with those classes of patients. Enrolling patients in clinical trials begins with the premise that these patients will achieve greater functional mobility through sessions of neuromuscular feedback therapy. Beginning with data gathered during clinical trials and, should they prove effective, regular sessions of neuromuscular feedback therapy, engineers make adjustments to the software algorithms and hardware mechanisms underlying the HAL suit, leading to yet more functional improvements in the robotic exoskeleton itself or even a new subtype of HAL suit optimized for the treatment of a particular kind of disability or disease. Patients, therapists, exoskeleton, engineers, and managers, then, are not just assembled together in space but are entangled temporally as the potential functionality of bodies and machines expands iteratively over time.

There is always the possibility that a clinical trial will fail. But it is precisely moments of failure that are seen to be the source of technological innovation. This is in part why the operation of the suit is monitored in real time. Without tracking moments of failure with actual patients, it would be harder to optimize the operation of the HAL suit for actual use, beyond what is achievable, say, with faster processor speeds or stronger component parts. What emerges is an entire economy of iterative engagement that extends beyond operational interactions between patients and the HAL suit in Germany, beyond the intense engagements of patients and therapists, to include computer servers in Japan, the decisions of the Federal Joint Committee in Germany, and, ultimately, the application of HAL technology to greater numbers of patients in Germany and beyond.

HAL is similar to Japanese care robots like AIBO and Paro in its harnessing of feedback as a therapeutic mechanism and in its mediation of interactions between care staff and patients. However, it differs from those animaloid robots both in form—it looks nothing like an animal—and in purpose. HAL aims for the incremental restoration of functional mobility, even if the path toward restoration proceeds through the brain. In targeting the physical needs of individuals who are not exclusively older adults, HAL is emblematic of a new generation of care robots that address more than the psychological needs of older adults with dementia. These "care robots 2.0" aim to support the physical demands of caring for others and everyday acts of living that older adults perform for themselves. It is to a discussion of these technologies that the next chapter turns.

SIX

Care Robotics 2.0 Meets Society 5.0

At the end of September in 2017, I took a train from central Tokyo to attend the 44th International Home Care and Rehabilitation Exhibition (HCR) at Tokyo Big Sight, a sprawling convention center near Tokyo Bay. HCR is an international exhibition for companies that sell products and services for older adults and people with disabilities. The exhibition in Japan is one of three held each year (the other expos take place in Europe and North America). HCR in Japan, a representative of the sponsoring organization told me, is typically the largest. Over three days, it draws around 120,000 attendees who visit booths displaying over 20,000 products from more than a dozen countries. At HCR 2017, conglomerates like Honda, Toyota, Mitsubishi, Panasonic, Toshiba, and Hitachi took pride of place among smaller companies from Japan, businesses from neighboring countries in Asia, and an assortment of European and American firms.

Visiting a product exhibition can be disorienting. There is the sheer enormity of the exhibition hall itself. There are the rows of brightly decorated booths. There are exhibitors shouting sales pitches over loud promo videos. Groups of visitors meander through narrow walkways, suddenly swarming to peek at items of interest. Yet what appears chaotic on the surface obeys the familiar logic of the market. Certain products—the newest—are featured;

certain features—the most desirable—are emphasized. Similarity in features drives the classification of products; classification takes tangible form in the spatial arrangement of exhibitors. In this way, product expos render visible a moment of economic activity. As one might study an art museum to learn how a society expresses history and identity through visual culture, one can observe at a product expo a market sector in material form.

I visited product exhibitions several times over years of research on care robots. Early on, I felt overwhelmed by the variety of technology and the sheer amount of information. At HCR 2017, though, I found myself much less bewildered than before. I recognized many of the firms and technologies and even knew some of the product representatives by name. I encountered familiar machines, Paro and HAL, surrounded by groups of visitors. But I also noticed a shift in the landscape of care robotics, driven in part by new priorities in healthcare and technology policy. Japan had begun moving beyond care robotics 1.0—the initial entry of robots into nursing care—toward care robotics 2.0, the roboticization of care technology itself.

Evidence of this shift was everywhere at HCR 2017, but it was hard to identify at first. For starters, the devices of care robotics 2.0 look different from their previous iteration. While robots emblematic of care robotics 1.0 are cute and cuddly like AIBO and Paro, and even the HAL exoskeleton approximates a human form, the robots of care robotics 2.0 look more like ordinary machines than living things. They also differ in purpose. Whereas the machines of care robotics 1.0 are employed in therapy for the body or mind, the devices of care robotics 2.0 assist with the labor of caring for others or the accomplishment of everyday life activities by older adults or people with disabilities. They also depend much more on constant network connections to external sensor and processing systems, making them hard to distinguish from consumer-oriented smart devices or even to classify together with the relatively autonomous machines of care robotics 1.0. What care robotics 1.0 tried to enclose in one discrete body, care robotics 2.0 instead distributes across a built environment of sentient machines.

In this chapter, I begin by reading HCR 2017 as a museum of care robotics 2.0. In the process of introducing these machines, I show how they emerged out of the same kinds of iterative encounters of users and makers that characterized care robotics 1.0. Like care robotics 1.0, they developed in response to policies that aimed to foster the development and promotion of robotics technologies for the aging society. Technologically, I argue further, iterative engagement has moved care robotics 2.0 toward what I call "thingification." Thingification openly embraces a machine aesthetic that fits robotics technology inconspicuously into care sites by adopting the look of other assistive technologies. It also offloads functionality onto human helpers or external machines, leading to a simplification of onboard features in the service of greater real-world efficacy. Care robotics 2.0 thus embraces what previously took technical know-how and tinkering to accomplish.

These shifts in form and function are reflected in new terminology. Instead of the care robots *(kaigo robotto)* I encountered in my initial fieldwork in Japan, care robotics 2.0 is populated by "robotic care devices" *(robotto kaigo kiki)*. These are machines that make use of robotics components but are not fully autonomous robots themselves. They often depend on an infrastructure of smart and sentient things. They thus manifest in form and function a trend toward the distribution of feeling—the capacity to sense and respond that I have considered distinctive of care robotics—across a range of connected technologies. As thingified robots, robotic care devices resonate with, even anticipate, the smart and sentient things of Society 5.0, a Japanese government vision of the future in which social life is facilitated by abundant feeling machines. This is not coincidental. The imagination of Society 5.0— the future as iteration, filled with feeling machines—is one shaped in part by a roboticist who put iterative engagements of humans and machines at the center of care.

Encountering Care Robotics 2.0

I might have missed many examples of care robotics 2.0 at the expo had I not looked at the products grouped under the subject heading "Robots" in the exhibit guidebook. I would surely have passed by Sasuke, which its manufacturer calls a "Robotic Care Device for Transfer Assistance." Sasuke looks more like a hydraulic lift on wheels than it does a conventional autonomous robot. The bottom portion of Sasuke has two wheeled "legs" that extend perpendicularly from a narrow base measuring about two feet high; its upper portion has two extensions on either side that function like arms. The upper section can be raised, lowered, or tilted from side to side (figure 6.1). Sasuke is intended to be used for "transfer," the movement of a person from one location to another. To transfer someone from bed to wheelchair, Sasuke's arms are lowered to mattress height and then inserted into a specially designed sheet that has been placed under the person. The care worker can then slowly raise Sasuke to lift the person from the bed and then angle them gently into a wheelchair.

Facilitating transfer qualifies Sasuke as a care device. Transfer aids are common in Japan and around the world, but they usually are fixed to ceiling tracks and function in only one area. Like these ceiling harnesses, Sasuke takes the burden of transfer off the body of a care worker (in fact, many countries have policies against care workers doing any lifting that is unassisted). However, it is mobile in a way that harnesses are not. Sasuke's purpose as a care device made sense when I visited the booth for its manufacturer, Muscle Corporation. Its status as a *robotic* care device was less obvious.

I asked a representative at the booth what made Sasuke a *robotic* care device. He replied that, according to the official government definition, as long as a machine is equipped with a sensor, a processing unit, and actuators, it can be called robotic. In Sasuke, all three processes (sensing, processing, acting) occur within the motors that make the machine move. Muscle Corporation calls these smart actuators "cool muscle" motors. The representative

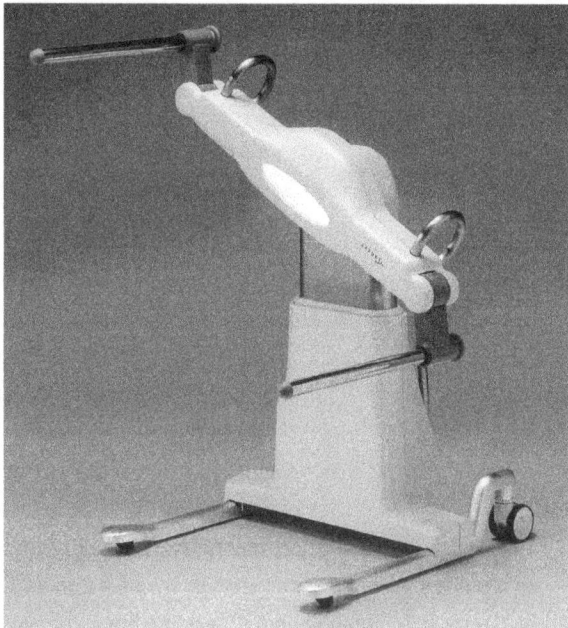

FIGURE 6.1 Sasuke.   Used by permission of MuscleCorp.

added that the company initially planned for Sasuke to determine the weight of the person being transferred and then move them between locations autonomously.[1] However, in the process of testing Sasuke in care facilities and listening to feedback from care staff, the company shifted direction. Rather than adding technological features just because they could, the company iterated in a new way. They reduced features in the service of greater functionality.

Not far from the Sasuke exhibit, the result of a similar development process was on display at the Panasonic booth. Panasonic's "Transfer Assistance Robot Resyone Plus" (hereafter, Resyone) is a combination bed and wheelchair the company has been developing for over a decade. At first glance, guard rails on each side of Resyone make it look like the kind of bed one might see at a hospital or nursing home. Unlike a typical bed, however, the Resyone divides lengthwise into two separate halves, with one half converting into a fully functional wheelchair. A care worker can transfer a person in the bed by raising the top half of the bed upward while simultaneously lowering the bottom half. They can then push the person as they would any other wheelchair.

This combination bed and wheelchair was similar in concept, yet different in final form, from a prototype that I saw at Panasonic's Osaka headquarters six years earlier. Much like early versions of Sasuke, that prototype was more technologically ambitious. It had a canopy that arched over the bed. On its underside, there was an LED monitor displaying a graphic interface used to control devices on a home network or access the internet. The bed was equipped with sensors that would monitor the vital signs of the person in the bed and notify a care provider if they detected a sudden abnormality. Perhaps most significantly, once converted from a bed to a wheelchair, the prototype could be driven by the seated person themselves using a joystick on the armrest.

This prototype iterated on an even older version of a Panasonic-made transfer device that that looked like Sasuke but had an even stouter frame and bulkier arms. When they exhibited this early prototype to the public, care professionals told them flatly that they would never have room for such an imposing machine. They also expressed concern about how safely it would handle the delicate bodies of frail older adults and how comfortable they might feel in its grasp. To address these issues, Panasonic engineers jettisoned their preference for humanoid form factors and redesigned the machine. The transforming bed was the result of these efforts but it, too, soon ran into problems. When trialing it at hospitals and care facilities, they found that it was still too big to function in institutional settings. Expensive sensors and motors also made it hard to bring down the cost of the device to an afford-able range. They removed the canopy and its associated sensors. They also removed the electric motor from the wheelchair, making it function more like a conventional wheelchair. By reducing the number and variety of fea-tures, Panasonic ended up with a device that could operate safely within care facilities (Kajitani and Wakita 2017, 468). As a journalist for the Japanese *Nikkei* newspaper wrote in 2014, in an article describing the development of the device, "The era in which large Japanese electronics companies use care facilities as spaces to show off the sophistication of their proprietary technol-ogy is over. There is no trace of the robotic in Panasonic's convertible bed. This is now simply a care device *(kaigo kiki)*" (Miura 2014).

How, then, could the company continue to market the bed as robotic when I saw it three years later in 2017? Even on my earlier visit to the Panasonic showroom, my guide admitted that it might be hard to see what remained of the robotic in the prototype bed/wheelchair. The difficulty can be traced to an elision between conventional understandings of robots as discrete, autono-mous devices and the recent preference of both government and corporations in Japan to think in terms of the more expansive category of "robot technol-ogy" *(robotto gijutsu)*. As long as a machine uses some combination of technol-ogies [components] that are vital to the operation of a robot—(1) sensors that send signals to (2) processing units that activate (3) servomechanisms—then it can be considered a robot technology. Practically speaking, it is not even necessary for all three of these technologies to be functioning together within a discrete machine for it to be considered robotic. Panasonic and Muscle Cor-poration adopt this liberal definition of the robotic when marketing machines that use parts of their proprietary robot technologies.

Categorizing Sasuke and Resyone as care robots reflects a generous un-derstanding of what it takes to be a robot technology. So, too, does it depend on a shift in what it means to care with robots. These robotic care devices do mediate acts of care and they do target the bodies of older adults and persons with disabilities. However, they are not meant to provide psychological heal-ing or to supplement physical therapy. Their status as care devices derives from their primary role in assisting with the labor of caring for others. Sasuke and Resyone express central elements of care robotics 2.0. They do not look like conventional humanoid or animaloid robots; in fact, it is challenging to understand how they are robotic at all. They work not autonomously but in conjunction with the movement of human bodies. They help people care for people, whereby caring means assistance with the performance of everyday physical acts, not relieving psychological distress or improving functional health. They also emerge through relations of corporations, care providers, and care recipients, iterative engagements that lead toward the simplification of features rather than increased complexity. Simplifying bulky machines that manipulate frail human bodies makes sense from the standpoint of safety; it reduces the likelihood of operator error or of injury from a random malfunction. But simplification also affects understandings of care robots themselves. They appear as discrete machines distinguished only by the use of a subset of vital robotics technologies or, as I show later, they become material nodes in distributed networks of sensors, processors, and actuators.

Hug, a transfer-assistance robot manufactured by Fuji Corporation, is an example of the former. Hug looks like a pint-sized version of Sasuke, with two padded arms that extend out from a control unit set atop a wheeled platform. To operate Hug, a care worker first wheels the machine in front of a seated person. The person then leans toward Hug, steps onto the platform, and hangs each arm over an arm pad. It is from this position, which makes it look as if the person is being embraced by the robot, that the machine gets its name. The care worker then uses a remote control to slowly raise the arms of the Hug and move the person into a standing position. Once secured in position, the carer can push Hug like a wheelchair to position the person in front of a chair, a toilet, or other object. Reversing these movements completes the transfer.

Like Sasuke and Resyone, Hug is intended to make the work of caring for others easier on the bodies of care workers. Yet, aside from the use of the word in its marketing materials, its status as a robot technology is not obvious. Hug certainly does not look like a conventional robot. Fuji claims that the machine operates on the basis of technologies borrowed from its own line of industrial robots.[2] Although it does not detail how (presumably it uses the same actuators as the company's industrial robots), the utilization of existing robotics technology is sufficient grounds for the company to call Hug a robotic care device.[3]

Not all newer care robots reapply technology borrowed from industrial robots. The cumbersomely named HAL Lumbar Type for Care Support uses the same feedback technology as the HAL lower-body exoskeleton, and is also worn around the waist. But it is designed for able-bodied adult care workers, not frail elderly or persons with disabilities (figure 6.2). When activated, the machine senses whether the wearer intends to bend down or up and provides assistive torque to reduce lower-back strain when lifting. It is also equipped with WiFi technology that enables real-time tracking of the machine's operation. The fact that it is wearable, rather than merely operated by a care worker, distinguishes the HAL Lumbar Type from transfer-assistance devices like Sasuke, Resyone, and Hug. Otherwise, it is similarly intended to reduce the physical strain of caring for others.

At HCR 2017, the HAL lower-body exoskeleton, which was much heralded when I began my fieldwork several years earlier, appeared less prominently that the HAL Lumbar Type. The Cyberdyne booth did feature a demonstration of the lower-body exoskeleton, but the amount of interest it attracted paled in comparison to the newer model. Each of the many times I passed by the Cyberdyne booth, I saw multiple people trying it out and others enthusiastically talking about it. I observed the same focus on the HAL Lumbar Type at a nearby booth for Daiwa House's care robot project. At the time, Daiwa House distributed both Cyberdyne's lower-body exoskel-

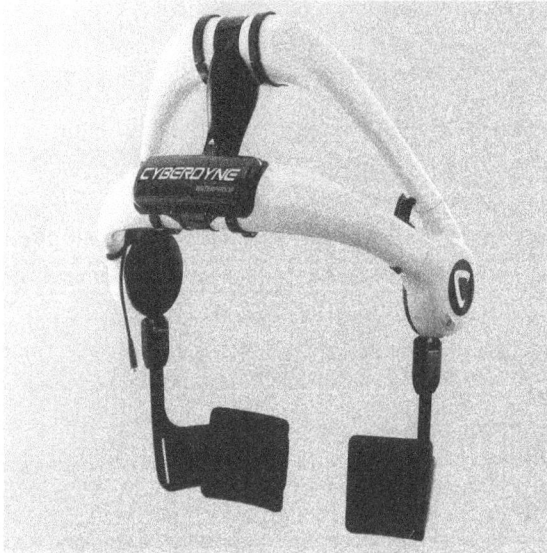

FIGURE 6.2 HAL Lumbar Type for Care Support.   Used by permission of CYBERDYNE Inc.

eton and lumbar-support device, yet only the lumbar-support robot appeared on display and in promotional literature.[4]

Visitors to both Cyberdyne's and Daiwa House's booths were likely most interested in robotics products that were approved by the Japanese government as nursing care devices and hence reimbursable under Japan's long-term care insurance system. The lumbar type had this certification while the lower-body exoskeleton did not. This made the lumbar-type model more appealing to institutions looking to reduce the likelihood of physical injury to their employees while containing costs. A Daiwa House representative provided an additional business rationale. Since it targets the healthy bodies of care workers, not just persons with walking disabilities, the lumbar type had many more potential users.[5] The iteration of HAL technology demonstrates how closely government insurance schemes are entangled with the profit-maximization strategies of corporations, in a way that does not necessary advantage older adults or persons with disabilities. It also illustrates how flexibly the notion of care can be interpreted. The HAL Lumbar Type is purportedly a technology built to manage the needs of caring for an aging society—the same rationale underlying the creation of the HAL lower-body exoskeleton. Frail older adults might indeed benefit from its use, but easing the labor of caring for the elderly and disabled is a very different aim than enabling them to care for themselves.

This is not to say that care robotics 2.0 entirely excludes robotic care devices for older adults themselves. HCR 2017 did feature mobility devices for older adults to use indoors and outdoors. Keipu and Rodem, for example, are made by two different companies that each reimagine the wheelchair along similar lines. Although Keipu is made by Fukushima-based Aizuk Corporation and Rodem by Kyūshū-based Tmsuk, both companies happen to use the same advertising tagline: "From cradling to riding piggyback" *(dakko kara onbu e)*. The terms *dakko* and *onbu* are Japanese words for carrying a child, either by cradling them in one's arms or by putting them on one's back. The marketing phrase suggests that the former is perceived to be more infantilizing for older adults than the latter. The agentive act of "riding" signals liberation from the passivity of being cradled by a wheelchair, whether motorized or not. Both machines are driven like scooters. In fact, Rodem looks like a scooter with two oversized wheels on each side. Keipu looks more like a padded lectern on wheels. Their seats and handlebars can be raised or lowered to facilitate getting on or off, performing a particular activity (e.g., washing hands), or raising oneself to the eye level of someone walking next to you.

Tmsuk and Aizuk both claim that these machines make it easier to care for older adults or for older adults to care for themselves. The ability of each machine to change shape is presented as a means of facilitating transfer (e.g., from bed to bathroom) and mobility (e.g., moving from one part of a residence to another). Yet, like other products distinctive of care robotics 2.0, it is not obvious what makes either machine robotic. Representatives for both companies remarked that the ability of their machines to change shape was important to their status as robots. They also stated that each machine borrows technologies engineered for other robots that each company manufactures. Rodem and Keipu are restricted to indoor use, and that likely accounts for their relatively simple features and functions. The unpredictable nature of outdoor settings requires more complex systems to manage.

Robot Assist Walker RT.1, and its lighter-weight successor RT.2, are examples of robotic care devices engineered for use outdoors. They look like wheeled walkers but are full of electronic components that provide greater functionality than a typical walker. Sensors in their handlebars measure the grip strength and walking speed of the person holding them. Additional motion sensors monitor the angle of the walker relative to the road as well as the condition of the road surface. Continual feedback from these sensors enables the walker to provide powered assistance. They also apply a braking mechanism automatically if a user's hands slip off the walker. The walkers can wirelessly connect to the internet and are also outfitted with GPS technology. Through wireless connection, they track calories expended, records walking distance and other mobility metrics, and accesses additional cloud services. Perhaps more controversially, an onboard GPS system permits a walker to be tracked, in case a family member wants to check on the status of the person walking with it. (It also can send an emergency alert to a designated contact person if there is sudden loss of contact with its handlebars.) Compared to other robotic devices at HCR, RT.1 fits squarely within the conventional definition of the robotic; it senses, processes, and activates servomechanisms that act in the physical world.

The kinds of robotic care devices displayed at HCR 2017 range considerably in their use of robotic components. Some, like Keipu and Rodem, use a subset; others, like the HAL Lumbar Type and RT.1, use all three. They differ as well in their target users, whether these be care recipients of care providers. Yet they share the same aim: to support the bodies of their target users.

Unlike the robots discussed in previous chapters, they do not target human bodies for therapeutic purposes or to enhance functional health. Their purpose is not repair; it is maintenance. They assist their users in performing the tasks of everyday life. This is not just a matter of applying robotics technology to new purposes. These robotic devices also look different from care robots like Paro and AIBO. In fact, they look much more like machines than living beings. There is no possibility of confusing, for example, Sasuke for a person with outstretched arms or of mistaking RT.1 for a guidance animal. Functionalist design aesthetics and simpler operation make these devices safer to use. While they operate in intimate, if not direct, connection with human bodies, they do not need to redirect attention to affect state of mind. They do not need to become companions or to mediate ties of affiliation in a field of human relations. They appear content to be things.

In the remainder of this chapter, I explore the reasons why care robotics 2.0 robots look and function as they do. I suggest that this is in part due to changing understandings of caring with robots that have been driven by shifts in healthcare policy. It is also partly due to a change in science and technology policy in Japan, one rooted in the modality of iterative development that has generated momentum for what I call the "thingification" of care robotics.[6] This policy promotes a vision of future technology where nearly all digital technologies people encounter are enrolled in processes of sensing, processing, and acting. The thingification of care robotics observable at HCR 2017 intersects with a government view of the future of technology in which all things digital have become more or less roboticized. In this future vision, iterative processes of feedback organize sociotechnical life and drive cycles of innovation. Such processes underlie the development of many of the robotic care devices I saw at HCR 2017. Perhaps more surprising, the policy vision itself has been shaped by the example of care robotics and by one of the pioneers in the field.

Care Robotics 2.0 for the Aging Society

In 2013, the Japanese Ministry of Economy, Trade, and Industry (METI) launched a program to develop and promote the adoption of "robotic care devices" *(robotto kaigo kiki)*. The impetus for this program, as for many previous projects related to care robotics, was Japan's aging society; specifically, the increasing need to support older adults and those who care for them in anticipation of population aging. Formally titled the Project to Promote the Development and Introduction of Robotic Devices for Nursing Care (in Japanese, *robotto kaigo kiki kaihatsu dōnyū sokushin jigyō*; hereafter, Care Robot Project), the initiative aimed to overcome perceived barriers to the rapid adoption of care robots by identifying the most significant needs of workers in the care field, setting safety standards and testing protocols for care robots, and providing financial support for developing care robots in line with funding priorities.[7] This included the establishment of a new independent administrative agency, the Japan Agency for Medical Research and Development (AMED), to oversee the project. The creation of AMED streamlined the regulation of new robotic care technologies, a bureaucratic process previously handled by three separate government ministries.[8] AMED seems like an answer to the frustrations of roboticists I met years early in my fieldwork who bemoaned the difficulties of navigating Japan's bureaucracy just to develop and test their technologies (see chapters 1 and 2). However, AMED and the Care Robot Project are not merely responses to the frustrations of robot inventors and manufacturers. By setting priority areas of development, they significantly direct the iteration of robotic care devices. They do not determine in advance what specific devices ought to be created, but they do establish market incentives and structure the regulatory context in which iterative engagements of robot makers and robot users unfold.

The Care Robot Project prioritized five categories of robotic care devices, each associated with a particular care need: (1) transfer aids (wearable and nonwearable); (2) mobility aids (outdoor and indoor); (3) toileting aids; (4) bathing aids; and (5) monitoring systems (for institutions and homes).[9] With the exception of monitoring systems, these areas map directly onto standard clinical metrics of functional health called "activities of daily life" (ADL). ADL—actions like moving one's body from place to place (transfer), going to the bathroom (toileting), cleaning oneself (bathing)—are believed by practitioners of biomedicine to be fundamental to everyday human life (Katz et al. 1963). ADL are used clinically as indicators of functional health, indexing the capacity of a person to live with a chronic health condition, disability, or other effects of physical decline. Indeed, when setting these priority areas, the Care Robot Project relied on a standard classification of disability and functional health used by the World Health Organization.[10] Conceptually, this connects the development of care robotics in Japan with global metrics of clinical medicine. More practically, it lends the project the imprimatur of a respected global health organization, making the products it supports more attractive to potential buyers at home or abroad. Such products include technologies for older adults or their helpers to use in carrying out everyday tasks. The Care Robot Project makes explicit what may have only been assumed in earlier perspectives on care robotics in Japan; namely, that care robots can support the bodies of care providers as well as those who qualify for care support under global metrics of functional health.

It is hard to overstate the impact of this project on the landscape of care robotics in Japan and on what I saw at HCR 2017. All of the aforementioned care robots fall into a priority area of the project, either as transfer aids (Sasuke, Resyone, HAL, Hug) or mobility aids (Rodem, Keipu, RT.1). All but two, Rodem and Keipu, received development subsidies from the project and feature prominently in its promotional materials. In addition, all were trialed extensively in actual contexts of care as part of their development process. (In fact, like Paro and the HAL lower-body exoskeleton, Rodem and Reysone were trialed abroad in Denmark before being sold commercially in Japan.)[11] Two of these devices—RT.1 and Hug—have released new versions of their robots in direct response to feedback from actual users even after first being commercialized. Perhaps even more important, all of these machines, even those that did not receive development funding from the project, are eligible for purchase or rental under Japan's LTCI. The official status of these technologies as "robotic care devices" *(robotto kaigo kiki)* contrasts with the representative machines of care robotics 1.0. Indeed, until a revision of the priority areas in 2017, AIBO, Paro, and the HAL lower-body exoskeleton would not have qualified for support under the project. Even after this revision, only Paro qualifies for inclusion in a newly established category of "communication robots" *(komyunikēshon robotto)*.[12]

Thingified Care Robots

It is uncertain whether the newest iterations of care robots, with their robust regulatory infrastructure and official support under the LTCI, will be more widely adopted than their predecessors.[13] What's clearer is that they have begun to change the prevailing image of Japanese care robotics. They look nothing like the humanoid robots imagined in the past to populate future robot towns (see chapter 2). Neither are they autonomous or multifunctional in the way robots of the future were once depicted. Care robotics 2.0 has been shaped less by the fancies of roboticists than it has by the expressed preferences of those for whom they are intended. Iterative engagements of users and makers yielded robotic care devices that are functionally simpler and relatively indistinguishable from ordinary things. Roboticists once thought that they needed to design machines that looked and acted familiar in order to avoid disrupting the flow of social life in the future. Instead, now years into the future once imagined, it might even be difficult for some to identify the thingified robots in their midst!

Thingified robots include machines like Sasuke and Hug that supplement physical acts of care and depend on a human operator. They also include devices that target the bodies of older adults but are not built to manipulate them or to generate a therapeutic effect. These robotic technologies are smaller in size than robots meant for transfer assistance or mobility. They also operate differently—they depend on a constant connection to the internet. In essence, they function only as material nodes in distributed networks of sensing and processing that facilitate the work of caring for others. Though new, in mediating networks of technologies and human care providers, these robotic things evoke older, mediated practices of caring with robots like AIBO and the HAL exoskeleton.

A machine I saw at Daiwa House's booth, the Silhouette Monitoring Sensor *(shiruetto mimamori sensā*; hereafter, Silhouette), is an example. Silhouette belongs to a priority category of robotic care device designated by AMED as "*mimamori robotto.*" These robotic care devices monitor the physical well-being of older adults discreetly. Silhouette itself looks like a miniature version of the ductless air-conditioning units that are common in Japanese households. It installs in a room high on a wall near the ceiling, and is equipped with a camera that points down at the bed and floor below it. When activated, Silhouette generates a two-dimensional monochrome image of a person's body position without displaying any identifying details. The person is effectively rendered in silhouette, a privacy feature and the origin of the device's name. The machine wirelessly transmits image data to the tablet or smartphone of a care worker or family member. Silhouette's vision sensors qualify it for inclusion as a robotic care device, but it is functionally useless without wireless connections to other internet-enabled technologies. According to the company that makes Silhouette, the machine can help nursing home staff keep tabs on residents without physically having to enter their rooms. Yet this value only emerges through a distributed system of objects and persons.

Similar in principle to Silhouette is a monitoring system called Nemuri-Scan ("Sleep Scan"). NemuriScan tracks whether a person is sleeping but does so without the use of any imaging technology.[14] Instead, it works by means of a flat sensor that is placed under the top mattress of a bed. This sensor responds to minute changes in pressure (i.e., the presence or absence of a person lying on a mattress) and is even sensitive enough to measure the rate at which a sleeping person breathes. NemuriScan processes this information onboard and then sends it to smart devices that are monitored by carers. But like Silhouette, it functions only through vital connections to networked things.

Thingified robotic care devices that monitor physical states are not limited to sensing physical presence. D-free, a wearable robotic care device supported by the Care Robot Project and displayed at Daiwa House's booth, senses when a wearer needs to urinate. From a belt around the waist, D-free sends ultrasonic signals into the bladder area. When these signals indicate that the bladder is full, D-free alerts a family members or care staff (not the wearer!) via smartphone notification. D-free can also track the timing and frequency of urination and automatically upload this information to care management software. These affordances qualify D-free for LTCI coverage as a "toileting aid" intended to save carers the expense of buying diapers and the time needed to manually record toilet habits. (Silhouette and Nemuri-Scan can also keep track of sleep rhythms.) In its critical connections to network technologies, D-free aligns with thingified robots like Silhouette and NemuriScan. In directly interfacing with care management system software, it demonstrates further how thingified robots can function dually by accomplishing individualized care and by automating the management of care work, a topic to which I will return.

Thingified robots that operate as nodes in networks of connected things are hard to confuse with conventionally humanoid or animaloid care robots. Yet, to my surprise, even the few humanoid care robots I encountered at HCR 2017 function as parts of distributed care systems. What struck me first about them was their size. In contrast to human-scale prototypes I had encountered in the past, these humanoid care robots were diminutive. Palro, an enthusiastically promoted humanoid robot made by Fujisoft, is only sixteen inches high; Sota, a robot distributed by the telecommunications company NTT Docomo, measures just under a foot. This small size reflects a change from the labor-saving duties imagined for humanoid robots in the past. These robots are instead meant to be placed on top of tables to serve as the focus of a group activity. They are officially classified as "communication robots," since they are equipped with voice recognition and speech synthesis technology. Promotional brochures for both robots, however, suggest that communication might not be their sole purpose within nursing homes. Both companies prominently feature photographs in brochures of these robots guiding groups of nursing home residents through exercise routines. Supporting "recreation" purportedly reduces the amount of time that staff have to spend getting their residents to move around and, obviously, raises the fitness levels of nursing home residents. The resemblance of this robot-guided activity to the way in which the Robot Therapy Group has used AIBO for years is striking (see chapter 3).[15] So, too, is the utilization of these robots to facilitate communication.

This functionality depends crucially on connections to external networking and processing technology. Sota, for example, can recognize voice commands and respond with synthesized speech but only after voice and speech data have been processed by NTT Docomo's "Roboconnect" cloud-service platform and transmitted back to the robot. This cloud platform also enables Sota to function as a real-time voice and image interface for video calls. Sota can also interface with internet-enabled, smart health technologies like blood-pressure monitors and temperature sensors as well as other smart home devices (Owada 2015). By adding yet another service ("Sota Rec"), the robot can be updated regularly with new exercise routines. These services are only available via subscription *after* renting or purchasing the robot. Robots arrive to a user, that is, lacking full functionality. The complete functionality of the robot emerges through connections to cloud services and other external technologies (at additional cost). When connected, Sota becomes at once more functional and less autonomous, more an embodied interface for the delivery of services than a discretely operational machine. Fujisoft, too, offers a subscription service that provides customizations for Palro (and revenue for Fujisoft). Platformizing robots is not entirely new—recall how the Robot Therapy Group platformized AIBO in an effort to enhance its functionality as a care device. In the case of these humanoid care robotics, however, platformization works through near-obligatory subscriptions. These monetize acts of caring with the robot in an ongoing way and, of course, also convert them into digital traces that can be logged and tracked. Digital data, in turn, becomes the basis for iterating devices in response to feedback from real-world operation. This demonstrates, as roboticists suggested to me early on in my fieldwork (and as I recount in chapter 2), that both monetization and miniaturization can be achieved by offloading aspects of the robotic—processing power, memory, voice recognition, speech production—onto machines located elsewhere. In so doing, care delivery becomes even more tightly entangled with centers of corporate power located far away, with humanoid robots functioning within distributed systems of internet-enabled things.

Humanoid care robots enmeshed in distributed networks like Sota and Palro, along with networked sensors like D-free and Silhouette, are good examples of what has come to be known as the "Internet of Things" (IoT). IoT was indeed a marketing buzzword at HCR 2017, where many machine makers touted internet accessibility and software companies advertised the ability of their cloud platforms to integrate digital data from multiple connected sources. The "efficiency" and "precision" that such automaticity purportedly provides for care workers is one of the merits of a software system sold by the company Good Tree. The company sells a temperature sensor, blood pressure sensor, activity monitor, and weight scale that automatically upload measurements to its proprietary cloud software system. This data can be recorded and tracked by care professionals, but this is only part of its value, according to the company. Older adults can keep track of their own health data, which the company says gives them "clear [health] goals [and] increased motivation to remain active," thus prolonging the time before nursing care becomes necessary (Good Tree, Corp. n.d.). The integration of vital sensing IoT devices and care management software also featured in promotional literature for a software platform sold by the company Kanamic, among others at HCR 2017. Care management systems might seem entirely distinct from care robotics, but such software platforms anticipated a revision to the Care Robot Project's list of priority areas that was announced the same month as HCR 2017. This revision expanded the areas of priority to include "devices that use robotics technologies to collect, store, and analyze data that assists in the provision of nursing care services for older adults" (METI 2017). The category includes monitoring and communication robots as well as software platforms, like those sold by Good Tree and Kanamic, that process the data they generate in real time. Whereas Sota and Palro are robots that have become to some extent platformized, care management systems offered by Good Tree and Kanamic are cloud software platforms that have become, officially at least, roboticized.

Judging by their promotional literature, the value of these software platforms lies primarily in their role as cloud-based tools to help manage the delivery of "community-based integrated care." Community-based integrated care *(chiiki hōkatsu kea shisutemu)* is a model of eldercare promoted by the Japanese central government since 2006 (Tsutsui 2014). Its intent is to overcome the fragmentation of eldercare across families, nursing homes, acute care centers, and welfare services by tightening the connections among them. Effectively coordinating action among this diversity of stakeholders demands considerable logistical and managerial support, which is precisely what these software packages promise. A marketing brochure from Kanamic, for example, illustrates how its "life-embracing cloud system" facilitates the sharing of information among doctors, home healthcare workers, nurses, pharmacists, volunteer workers, government care managers, and families (Kanamic n.d.). Seamless IT solutions aside, observers have noted how the community-based integrated care system represents a redistribution of responsibility for eldercare away from publicly supported health and welfare programs to entire communities (Tsutsui 2014, 4), a move made in an attempt to control the cost of an LTCI system that has increased by more than three times since its inception in 2000 (Yamada and Arai 2020, 175–76).

The emergence of care management platforms is significant not just for the way in which they technologically support the delegation of healthcare from state institutions to civil society. As much as cloud software systems might try to knit together fragmented communities of care, they depend on the fragmentation of robotics technologies that were once integrated. If care robotics 1.0 fetishized the effect of one-on-one engagement with an autonomous robot (even if such autonomy was in fact illusory), care robotics 2.0 eschews any pretense of autonomy and embraces the expansion of functionality afforded by distributed processing and sensor networks. Care management systems and their inclusion among the priority areas of the Robot Care Project are emblematic of this shift in thinking about the nature of robotics. This is a shift that has developed through iterative engagements of technology makers, care professionals, and care recipients, engagements that have produced things that act like robots and robots that look like things.

Robotic Care Devices and the Future Iterated

The thingification of care robotics reflects a broader governmental interest in roboticizing things even beyond the field of care. This interest is articulated forcefully in the national government of Japan's Science and Technology Fifth Basic Plan. A key aspiration of this policy that was effective from 2016 to 2021 is the realization of "Society 5.0," which is defined elsewhere in the plan as the "super smart society" *(chō sumāto shakai)*.[16] Outlined in the vague but nevertheless grandiose language of future-oriented policy documents, the super smart society is said to merge "physical space (real world) and cyberspace by leveraging ICT [information and communications technologies]" in order to create a "human-centered society that promotes economic growth while resolving social problems."[17] The super smart society depends further on developing the Internet of Things; that is, "the connection of 'things' which have so far functioned separately . . . into 'systems' using cyberspace . . . [in order to] realize an abundant and high quality of life for citizens" (Government of Japan 2016, 13).

Exactly which social problems need resolution is left less well-defined than the technologies that will purportedly power the super smart society of the future. It is a plan oriented toward science and technology after all. However, in a section detailing how Society 5.0 will marshal science and technology to achieve sustainable growth, the first social issues mentioned are aging and depopulation. Specifically, the policy states that developing advanced medical technology is vital to "handle hyper-aging [and] depopulation" and to "[establishing] a society in which people enjoy long and healthy lives." Doing so not only will help assuage the twin pressures of aging and depopulation, it also will improve "competitiveness in . . . medical related industry [and] contribute to our nation's economic growth" (Government of Japan 2016, 22). Concern about an aging society even finds expression in a section of the policy on securing a food supply for the future, where worries about a "[declining] and aging . . . labor force" are to be addressed through the promotion of " 'smarter' agriculture that utilizes ICT and robot technology to achieve lower costs and large-scale production" (Government of Japan 2016, 21). Although Society 5.0 is a new vision, the role of technology in solving intractable social problems, the place of the aging society as one of the foremost social problems, and the achievement of economic growth through the resolution of social issues resonate in the previous chapters of this book.

Society 5.0 owes a conceptual debt to the German plan for Industrie 4.0. But what the German plan limits to a project to improve the efficiency of manufacturing, the Japanese initiative iterates a step further to society itself. In the Japanese plan, iteration is not just a mechanism that can bring about technological innovation. It is metaphorical lens through which to understand the relationship between technological change and social transformation. In fact, policy documents prepared by the Cabinet Office, as well as the influential Japanese business federation Keidanren, reconceive the entire history of human civilization through the lens of iteration.[18] The period dating from the earliest evidence of modern humans to the emergence of the agricultural society in 13,000 BCE is called Society 1.0. Society 2.0 runs all the way from the dawn of agriculture to the industrial revolution in Europe. The first and second industrial revolutions bookend Society 3.0, or the industrial society, and the third industrial revolution heralds the beginning of the information society (Society 4.0) in the closing decades of the twentieth century. Society 5.0 lies at the terminus of this linear historical evolution and accompanies the digital technologies of the fourth industrial revolution like artificial intelligence, the Internet of Things, and blockchain technology. With the notable exception of Society 5.0, these epochs are symbolized and propelled by a particular technology: Society 1.0 by the bow and arrow; Society 2.0 by agricultural tools; Society 3.0 by the railroad and factory; and Society 4.0 by the desktop computer and later the smartphone. Society 5.0, by contrast, is represented by a cartoon character jumping for joy, an expression perhaps of the expected liberation of humans from work by technologies like AI and IoT.

Idealistic visions aside, iteration also underlies the operation of Society 5.0. The super smart society realizes its quality-of-life gains by means of continuous feedback between distributed networks of sensors and processing units. Sensors respond to the changes in human behavior and responses, convert these responses into digital data, and then send this data to processing systems that feed the information back as "value-added" information for humans and machines in the physical world.[19] In linking thingified robots—distributed sensors, processors, and actuators—Society 5.0 expands the model of distributed care robotics I saw at HCR 2017 into a total social vision. Care platforms fed by internet-connected sensing devices anticipate this model of human-centered systems of distributed technologies. I would argue further: by placing the sensing of human intention and behavior at the center of technological innovation, the robots of care robotics 1.0 and the thingified robots of care robotics 2.0 are paradigmatic expressions of the iterative mechanisms underlying Society 5.0. Think, for example, of the HAL exoskeleton with its trifold elaboration of the feedback principle as a means of machine operation, care delivery, and technological development. The seamless circulation of information between the physical body and digital machines has been a consistent feature across the many iterations of HAL technology.

HAL and Society 5.0

At first, I thought that similarities between the principles of HAL technology and the principles of Society 5.0 were just coincidence. When I learned more about the construction of the new policy, however, I found that one of the key intellectual architects of Society 5.0 was Prof. Yoshiyuki Sankai, inventor of HAL technology and CEO of Cyberdyne. To learn more, I met Prof. Sankai in fall 2017 to discuss Society 5.0 and new developments in HAL technology. He first minimized his role, portraying himself as a consultant who only helped develop key concepts used in the plan. He earned this consultancy not solely due to his many grants and headline-grabbing technologies but also because of his role as program manager for a Cabinet Office initiative to foster disruptive innovation. But as we progressed in our conversation and through a set of PowerPoint slides that he had prepared, it became clear that the thinking behind Society 5.0 reflected perspectives long held by Prof. Sankai, especially his vision of the relationship between human beings and digital technologies. "For a long time, the connection between the physical world and the world of information has been managed by industry," he told me. "That's what the plan calls Society 4.0, or Industrial Society. But there's something important missing from that vision of society—that's information about people *(hito no jōhō)*. Conceiving of robots and humans as part of the same information ecosystem has been my specialty for years, whether that be neurological information, physiological information, or physical information. This is why I took part in this plan. It emphasizes the information interface mediating things and people."

An "information interface mediating things and people" describes well the distributed care technologies that I saw at HCR 2017. These technologies extend the provision of care by sensing physical movement or the intention thereof, maintaining a connection to processing units located elsewhere, and later adding value to both carers and creators by storing and analyzing the digital traces of action in the physical world. Although they are categorized as "robotic care devices," they approach something more like a *system* than a discrete thing. This, too, aligns with Prof. Sankai's thinking. Throughout our conversation, he referred to his signature exoskeleton as "cybernic system HAL." Practically, when applying for research and development support, this allowed him to thread a bureaucratic line between agencies that back robotics projects and those that fund medical research. Symbolically, it marked something more; namely, a conception of his device as more than just a therapy robot that acts and reacts locally in response to changes in human bodies. Cybernic system HAL is a physical *interface* to the "space of digital information" *(jōhō kūkan)*. In contrast to my time at CCR, where connections between HAL exoskeletons in Germany and Cyberdyne servers in Japan went unstated until I inquired directly, Prof. Sankai described how fundamental network linkages were to his technology and the related technological vision of Society 5.0.

> We created a technology [HAL] that does more than respond to signals from the cerebral nervous system and achieve a therapeutic effect through constant feedback. By virtue of a physical connection to the exoskeleton, one is also connected to a larger computerized environment *(kankyō)*. This device—this cybernic system—is an interface. It transforms a local interaction in the physical world into data that is then sent to a supercomputer for processing. Everything is entangled, from the human–robot cybernic system to the supercomputer.

Prof. Sankai's description of HAL technology as an interface that positions human bodies in the physical world in an extractive relationship with distributed digital technologies expresses in microcosm the broader societal aims of Society 5.0. One need only think of the promotional image, referenced in the preface, of the multigenerational family encircled by overlapping technological loops. Yet the massive amount of data extracted by the HAL robot/interface, or collectively by the imagined devices of a Society 5.0, does not necessarily accrue to the benefit of any one individual under treatment. By definition, big data is data in the aggregate. And it is harnessed for the benefit of makers like Cyberdyne (and possibly, but not certainly, future users). HAL operates, then, much like other products of the fourth industrial revolution that "continue to gather [usage] data after [they] are sold" (Deguchi et al. 2020, 18). Continual data gathering, whether automated or not, is fundamental to both the iterative provision of care, the vision of Society 5.0, and the development of the care robots reviewed in this book. Robotic care devices are not the only kinds of digital technologies included under the umbrella of Society 5.0. But in the primacy of sensing and responding to human bodies, in the intimacy of their skin-to-surface operation, in their placement of the human at the center of connected digital technologies in the service of technological development, they are emblematic of its aims, if not, as in the figure of Prof. Sankai, of direct influence on its conception.

Coda: Cybernic City

In our conversation, Prof. Sankai slipped easily between talking about his company's products and the technologies underlying Society 5.0, so much so that at times it was hard for me to see where the aims of Cyberdyne ended and the aspirations of Society 5.0 began. After our interview concluded, I walked down to the lobby of the Cyberdyne headquarters. There I saw a wall-sized display panel with an image that made clear this was not accidental. Printed at the top of the panel, under the Cyberdyne corporate logo, were the words "Society 5.0: Social Innovation by Innovative Cybernic Systems." The rest of the panel, which was written entirely in English, was divided into two sections. On the left, under the heading "Cybernic Interface/Device," were an assortment of Cyberdyne technologies—the HAL lower-body exoskeleton, its lighter-weight cousin meant for supporting the lower backs of workers, and a range of wearable, vital sensing devices. At lower right was a small overhead view of a lived community drawn like a cartoon, with homes, streets, a park, a shopping mall, and a hospital. On the periphery of the town was a modern, multistory office building with the name "Cyberdyne Social Innovation Base." From devices on the left and scenes of everyday life activities on the right, dashed lines arched toward the Social Innovation Base, where they terminated in directional arrows (figure 6.3).

This representation of unidirectional flow surprised me. In contrast to the images of care technologies I had encountered previously, including even the video of the HAL exoskeleton that ran on repeat on an LED screen next to this display, visualizations of feedback between humans and machines featured much more prominently than arrows of linear directionality. As lines arched toward a technology from a person, other lines would typically wind back from the technology toward the person. These illustrate the typical feed-back loop—the iterative cycle—that I have followed throughout this book. But here, perhaps unintentionally, that loop had been broken. The arrows only flowed one way, toward a center of corporate technology development. Through these flows, as the panel made explicit and Prof. Sankai had re-marked in our conversation, the center gathered "big data on physical, physi-ological, and life information." It may have been that the feeding back of this data into devices was assumed to be implicit in the language of "social inno-vation." Or, perhaps, the panel belied the fundamentally extractive nature of Cyberdyne's many cybernic interfaces.[20] Perhaps the same, too, can be said of Society 5.0, appearing here in direct alignment with the Cyberdyne brand.

The depiction of community life entangled in a cybernic system reminded me of a new project Prof. Sankai mentioned in our conversation. His business had recently purchased land a few minutes' drive from its corporate head-quarters in Tsukuba City with the intention of building "Cybernic City." Cy-bernic City would house a number of organizations focused on the innovation of new technologies for Cyberdyne as well as a hospital, presumably where these technologies could be applied. Of greater significance, the city was to

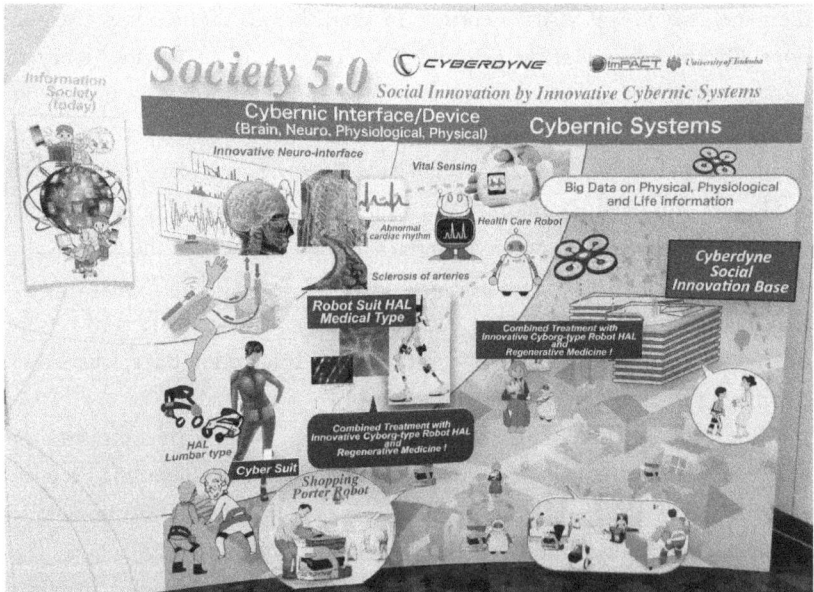

FIGURE 6.3 Cyberdyne Inc. and Society 5.0.   Photo by author.

include a state-of-the-art living facility for older adults, a "Technopia Support Community." Rather than rely on outside hospitals or nursing hospitals to furnish test sites for its products, Cyberdyne would in essence build its own.

This was only a plan that might or might not happen, Prof. Sankai cautioned. The note of caution about the unpredictability of what the future might bring, along with a well-organized set of PowerPoint slides detailing a techno-utopian urban solution to the problems of an aging society, brought me back to another slideshow and another urban plan for the aging society: Robot City CoRE and the presentation of Dr. Kagawa with which this book opens. That failed project and Prof. Sankai's planned project—one could add as well, the social vision of Society 5.0—share in the desire to solve the problems of older adults in the future. In Cybernic City, the crisis of aging society appears yet again, serving once more to legitimate the pursuit of new technologies. What seems rarely accounted for is whether technologies accomplish the goal of helping actual older adults. Would the Cybernic City ever be built? If it were, would it be yet another ground for creating technologies that develop, through multiple iterations, away from the target audience of older adults who provide vital feedback along the way? Ultimately, it seemed to me, the process—the urge to develop, to ceaselessly iterate—was the point.

I asked Prof. Sankai about the specific framing of this future in terms of the iterative modalities of Society 3.0, 4.0, and 5.0. I expected him to mention the reliance of Society 5.0 on new information and communications technologies. His answer was even more instructive, and reflective of the aims of this book. "Why 5.0, you ask? Well, the 'point zero' means this is not a digital on or off, like a one or zero. It means continuous change. A little bit up, an increment. We are here now, and after Society 5.0, maybe there comes a Society 5.1 . . ."

Addicted to the Future

In October 2017, a few days after talking with Prof. Sankai at Cyberdyne, I arranged to visit the Muratas, the couple whose upstairs room I rented in Tokyo during my fieldwork seven years earlier. The subway ride took me across town to a familiar stop. A wave of nostalgia passed over me as I retraced the steps to a place that I had once known so well. Keiko Murata greeted me at the door, and invited me to join her at a table in the center of their living room. This is where I would always sit when I visited the couple in the past, since it was right next to Minoru Murata's bed. Where the bed used to be, there was now a small couch. I felt terrible about not having been in better touch. Minoru had passed away four years earlier.

Keiko told me what happened. One day, Minoru spiked a high fever. His doctor prescribed a course of antibiotics, but the fever did not subside. When it spiked again, they rushed to a large hospital nearby by ambulance. He was admitted but the cause of his symptoms could not be confidently determined. Tests suggested that Mr. Murata had been aspirating food into his lungs, which in turn had brought on pneumonia. Hospital staff restricted his diet to jello, which seemed to reduce his fever. He was discharged after a month with instructions to remain on a strict diet. Only a few weeks later, though, his symptoms returned. He was hospitalized again, now in a much weaker state because of his limited calorie intake. He never recovered.

The experience left Keiko frustrated by the quality of care they had received and without a partner with whom she had shared most of her adult life. She preferred talking about their good times together. They first met at a pharmaceutical company in Tokyo, he a fresh college graduate and she a recent arrival to the city from the countryside. Giggling, she recalled their first few months together going to the movies and to amusement parks on dates. She spoke fondly of the years after Mr. Murata's retirement when they divided their time between Tokyo and a country cottage in Nagano Prefecture. She reminisced about their forty-four trips abroad, pictures of which they were always happy to show me when I visited with them in years past. Renting a room to overseas researchers helped them maintain a sense of the world beyond Japan even when travel became harder to manage in later life.

Mr. Murata never was able to take advantage of the HAL exoskeleton I had described to him many years before. HAL had developed into a device primarily for the rehabilitation of younger persons with disabilities (whom I describe in chapter 5), not older adults having trouble navigating homes and streets. His mobility had nevertheless improved since I first met him. Keiko told me that he had connected with a talented physical therapist before he got ill. Sessions with the therapist helped him recover more mobility. He could get up from bed, walk to the front door of their house with a cane, and navigate the step down from the floor to the wheelchair near the front door by himself. Outside, he could walk a short distance down their street and return again, stepping back into the house under his own power. He could also handle twice-a-week baths and eat a much more varied diet. It's hard to know how much more mobility he might have recovered had there been care robots that suited his needs. For Mr. Murata, "robotic solutions for the aging society" remained consigned to a future someday, a someday that never came.

As I progressed in my fieldwork in Japan, then Denmark, and then Germany, I kept Mr. Murata and others like him in my thoughts. Sometimes they became hard to see, invisibilized in the present for the sake of the elderly of the future whose "problems" would be solved by robotics technology. They rooted me in the present as I tracked the divergent trajectories of technologies purportedly meant to serve their needs now and into the future. They provided a counterpoint to the unblinking gaze toward the future so common among the roboticists I met. "Japanese are kind of addicted to the future," an engineer at Cyberdyne who had worked in both Germany and Japan told me. "The country has a lot of research funding for robotics but it's not just an issue of money. I'm always surprised when I see housewives visiting our showroom to check out HAL. That would almost never happen in Germany!"

Addicted to the future. Essentialist as it is, the engineer's turn of phrase struck me as insightful then and still does now. Its sentiment sits uneasily next to the urgent presentism that opens this book—Mr. Murata's demand that robotics companies "hurry up and make something I can use!" For people like Mr. Murata, futuristic technology promises an immediate remedy for a pathological condition. For those whom the engineer has in mind, the future is itself a fetish object of affective intensity bordering on the pathological. Failure to realize the future is a tragedy for those who need care now; it is a transitional step along the spiral path of innovation for those who make care machines.

———

This book has examined the work of caring with robots in three countries. In none of the sites it surveys do robots fully take over the human role in caring for others. Whether it be a group of aging engineers tinkering with AIBO in Japan, care workers in Denmark introducing Paro into interactions with nursing home residents with dementia, or physical therapists in Germany supervising patients walking with the exoskeleton HAL, robots mediate relations of care between and among people. They are in this way no different from other analog and digital technologies used within practices of care and that have much longer histories. By virtue of the capacity of these robots to respond to changes in emotional expression and behavior in real time, however, care workers and care recipients attribute to these feeling machines a powerful "feedback effect." These effects reverberate beyond moments of care to encompass both the makers of care robots and the researchers who study them. The effects of caring with robots, that is, are entangled with the continued technological development of care robots, shaping their material futures and the kinds of care relations they might afford into the future.

These iterative engagements, as I call them, unsettle distinctions of the laboratory and the field. They align in form and in purpose with the projects of an earlier generation of Japanese roboticists who saw the placement of experimental robots into everyday settings as crucial to the technological development of machines that could function successfully within them. Indeed, they undergird the vision of a future Japan running entirely on the basis of relations of feedback between humans and digital machines embodied by the government of Japan's plan for a future Society 5.0. Plans for the future aside, even more so than at the start of my research over a decade ago, it is difficult to imagine navigating daily life in the Global North (and increasingly in the Global South as well) without relying on digital technology—a daily life, that is, free from iterative engagement.

Looking back, it is hard not to register the influence of a particular set of economic circumstances during this same period. My research and writing overlapped with one of the longest stretches of sustained economic expansion in the United States through the 2010s, and the ongoing rise of China as a global economic power and partner in the high-quality, low-cost manufacture of cheap electronic components at scale—both coinciding with the anticipation that Prime Minister Abe's aggressive, multipronged economic stimulus plan for Japan (colloquially known as "Abenomics") would bring an end to post-Fukushima malaise. Through the mid-2010s, it seemed that each year would bring the steady iteration of ever-smarter technologies that promised upgraded features to users while servicing ever more information about users to corporate centers. Sale of these devices, the services they offered, and the digital ties they established proved highly valuable. Their global appeal catapulted American tech firms into positions of economic dominance, so much so that they came to be known collectively by the acronym FAANG (Facebook, Amazon, Apple, Netflix, Google). Japanese companies were not far behind in riding the wave of tech optimism, most notably Softbank, which acquired the humanoid robot Pepper from the French firm Aldebaran in 2014 and purchased the US-based leader in humanoid robotics Boston Dynamics in 2017 (Tilley 2017). The high-profile acquisition of Pepper—"the world's first personal robot that can read emotions"—and Boston Dynamics, a firm well known for sensational YouTube videos of its humanoid and animaloid robots dancing, jumping, and twisting with lifelike realism, symbolized not only the continued belief of Japanese in the promise of emotionally intelligent robots but also the investment of a major corporation in its realization.[1]

As many readers will surely know, complacency about a steadily expanding economy driven by the continuous iteration of digital technologies came to an abrupt end in 2020 as the COVID-19 pandemic spread across the globe. Lockdowns to suppress the spread of the coronavirus led to a precipitous drop in economic activity worldwide and to the disruption of global supply chains crucial to the mass production of consumer technologies. The physical confinement of lockdown, coupled with the admonitions of public health officials to "social distance" from friends and relatives, disrupted as well quotidian rhythms of life across the globe. For all but so-called essential workers, daily rituals of school, work, childcare—even mundane trips to grocery stores, restaurants, movie theaters, and sporting events—were upended.

Ordinary markers of social time having vanished, it became difficult to separate one day from another. In these darkest times of the pandemic, when death rates were soaring and a vaccine was still believed to be years away, the present seemed to have reached out and swallowed the future, such that people across the globe were all living in a perpetual meantime. In an essay entitled "Pandemic Time," the political scientist Alister Wedderburn expresses this shared experience well. "I am inhabiting the temporality of a dog," Wedderburn writes. "For the last fourteen weeks, my time has revolved around meals and once-daily walks. Everything else is mush" (Wedderburn 2020, 31).

Like Wedderburn, I, too, felt the mush of pandemic time. Many of the chapters of this book were composed or completed in the midst of the pandemic, and I felt viscerally a gap between the unbridled optimism for an anticipated future that runs through them and the dreary meantime suffusing my everyday life. I began to wonder whether the disruption so valued by proponents of iterative development had itself been brought to an end by a tiny virus. How much did spiraling relations of feedback between humans and machines matter when ordinary interactions been humans had been so critically undermined? Without a future to anticipate, what sense did iterative engagements make? Had our intimate connection to digital technologies been irreversibly severed?

Despite the lingering presence of the pandemic, these concerns turned out to be short-lived. The pandemic certainly did disrupt everyday social life. But its effect on everyday interactions with digital technology was far less clear. In my own work as an educator, previously niche digital software applications like Zoom and Microsoft Teams enabled me and my colleagues to continue teaching students, albeit in a radically different way than before. Fast broadband connections made it possible for multitudes of white-collar workers to forego commutes and to do work, which was already heavily reliant on computers and the internet, at home. Government meetings, court proceedings, medical appointments, and even fun meet-ups with friends went remote. In some countries, especially in East Asia, digital technologies were enrolled in the control of infections through mobile apps designed to track the expression of symptoms in local populations and to monitor their movements.[2] Suddenly, the experience of emotional connection, not to mention physical surveillance, afforded by digital technologies of sensing and response seemed far less confined to the fringes of care that I trace in this book. Engagements with such technologies were now much more broadly shared, enabling people to maintain sociality despite restrictions on physical movement, while also making possible forms of surveillance that previously would not have been so well-tolerated.

In Japan, the COVID-19 pandemic prompted a renewed commitment to the vision of Society 5.0 first articulated in the government's Fifth Science and Technology Basic Plan only a few years before. The government's successor plan—now named the Science, Technology, and Innovation Plan—outlines concrete steps toward the realization of Society 5.0, including an investment of 30 trillion yen ($224 billion) in research and development funding that the government hopes will serve as a "catalyst" for an additional 120 trillion yen ($824 billion) outlay by the private sector in support of the Society 5.0 vision (Cabinet Office of Japan 2021, 4). The COVID-19 pandemic did little to dissuade leaders in Japan from believing in the centrality of ubiquitous and responsive digital technologies to the country's future and economic vitality. By the middle of 2020, the government noted that "delay in the digitalization of Japan and . . . realization of Society 5.0 . . . has shackled efforts to prevent infection while also continuing corporate activities and social activities" (Cabinet Office of Japan 2020, 2). To overcome this delay, the government launched an effort to digitalize consumer and government services known by the moniker "digital transformation," or DX. The government passed a policy framework for DX in December 2020, and by September of the following year had established a brand-new Digital Agency to promote the digitalization of government and business activity. Without regard to the eventual success or failure of these measures, the commitment to both DX and Society 5.0 symbolizes an intensified effort to bring everyday activity in the public and private sectors into the fold of networked digital devices. Viewing the future through the lens of iteration, even with the challenges of a global pandemic, has seen little interruption in Japan. The same is true for the ever-serviceable crisis of the aging society. In fact, in its outline on the formation of a digital society, the government stresses that digitalization is "extremely important for responding to the rapidly declining birth rate and aging population" (Digital Agency 2021).

————

In June 2021, Softbank announced that it was pausing production of the humanoid robot Pepper (Tsuneoka 2021).[3] Despite claims about its advanced ability to perceive emotion, Pepper, which sold for approximately $2,000, did not persuade buyers that it could perform tasks like greeting customers and giving directions better (or more cheaply) than a human worker. Some nursing homes in Japan had also trialed Pepper to no avail (Vogt and König 2021), which makes the robot appear to be yet another failed attempt to introduce care robotics into Japanese nursing care. Of course, it could very well be that Pepper has reached the end of its operational life. Notably, however, Softbank only "paused" production of the robot. Could the company instead package its technology in a different, more salable form? It is too early to tell. And, I would suggest, too soon to call its underlying technology a failure. It could be that this is but one moment in the iteration of Pepper's technology, one inflection point that shifts the development trajectory of the robot in a new direction, whether toward the field of care or away from it. I would caution not to extrapolate too hastily from Pepper's widely reported demise to dismiss the future potential of robotics technology in care more generally. As I note in chapter 6, the category of robotic care devices in Japan is so flexible that is hard not to imagine some form of care robotics that will prove attractive at home or elsewhere.

Indeed, the focal technologies examined in this book have not gone the way of Pepper. The robot Paro continues to be used in the care of dementia in sites across the world, and its interactions with care workers and care recipients continue to spawn new potential applications. A newspaper recently reported, for instance, that Paro is being considered by NASA as a device that might provide stress relief on long spaceflights (Banno 2023). Cyberdyne Care Robotics continues to operate in Germany, and, following the approval of HAL as a medical device in Japan, feedback training with the lower-body exoskeleton has expanded to five locations in the country and abroad to eighteen additional countries.[4] Even the AIBO robot dog, which Sony discontinued in 2006, has found a new lease on life. Eleven years later, Sony released a new version. This iteration is intentionally platformized in a way reminiscent of its ad hoc platformization by the tinkerers of the Robot Therapy Group in Japan. Advanced features of the robot are only accessible via a subscription AI Cloud Plan that includes cellular coverage to maintain independent use of the robot outside of home wireless networks.[5] Connection to the cloud provides the new AIBO with a longer memory as well as an expanded capacity to learn and grow, thus entangling it in the same loops of feedback between users and makers distinctive of HAL and other examples of care robotics 2.0. Japan's digital push makes it likely that the robots of the future, the robots meant for yet another iteration of the future aging society, will be similarly entangled, despite the challenges they face in the present. The recent emergence and rapid adoption of generative AI systems like Open AI's Chat GPT, Google's Bard, and Microsoft's Copilot suggests that the platformized robots of the future might become even more capable than we can presently imagine. It remains to be seen just who will be included in that future and who will be left waiting for someday.

ACKNOWLEDGMENTS

Apropos of its subject matter, the chapters of this book went through many iterations before arriving at their present form. I benefited at every step from the generous feedback of colleagues and friends. Erik Love was a constant and cheerful interlocutor over the years of my research and writing. He offered insightful comments on all chapters, and I am filled with gratitude for his help. Anne Allison read every chapter of the draft manuscript and provided crucial insights that guided editing and revision. Jeffrey Bass, Laura Tubelle de González, and Akiko Takeyama reviewed chapter drafts and offered wonderfully constructive suggestions. An afternoon brainstorming session with Maria Toyoda helped bring the ideas underlying the manuscript into much sharper focus. The reports of anonymous reviewers for Stanford University Press helped me see again the manuscript holistically with fresh eyes. The book would not be what it is without the efforts of all of these individuals. Any errors or shortcomings that remain are, of course, entirely my own.

Parts of this book were presented to audiences at Temple University, the University of Tokyo, Harvard University, and the Nordic Institute of Asian

Studies, and I appreciate the engagement and generous provocations of those audiences. My thinking about this project has also been shaped over the years in conversation with Jason Karlin, Satsuki Takahashi, David Leheny, Stefan Tanaka, Marc Moskowitz, Jason Danely, Ryo Morimoto, Patrick Galbraith, Theodore Bestor, Andrew Gordon, Susan Long, David Jordan, Sharla Blank, Adrian Cruz, and Kazuyo Kubo.

My colleagues in East Asian studies Alex Bates, David Strand, Neil Diamant, Nan Ma, and Akiko Meguro graciously supported this project from inception and accommodated all of my requests for research leave to bring it to completion. My knowledge of issues related to aging benefited greatly from co-leading two student field-study programs on later life in the United States and Japan. Discussions with students, our interlocutors, and colleagues David Sarcone and John Henson deepened my knowledge of healthcare systems and health-related quality of life. I am grateful as well for the support and engagement over the years of other scholars and friends, including Evan Young, Wei Ren, Helene Lee, Jennifer Schaefer, Suman Ambwani, Andrew Wolff, Claire Seiler, John MacCormick, Kamaal Haque, Antje Pfannkuchen, Elizabeth Lee, Adeline Soldin, and Burleigh Hendrickson. Special thanks as well to Todd Arsenault for lending his considerable talents to the preparation of images and photos for submission.

It was a privilege to be invited into the lives of people whose voices, which remain anonymous for purposes of privacy, reverberate through these pages. I am indebted to the many roboticists I met in Japan who kindly shared their time and passion for their machines with me, especially the members of the Robot Therapy Group. I thank Takanori Shibata and Yoshiyuki Sankai, in particular, for granting my interview requests and for taking the time to talk with me, sometimes on multiple occasions. My research in Denmark would likely not have happened without the help of Christina Leeson, who provided crucial assistance when making initial contacts. Julie Munk and Anne-Lise Hansen arranged visits to nursing homes in and around Copenhagen, and I can't thank them enough for opening their lives as carers to me and for introducing me to the many older men and women whom they engage in their work. While in Denmark, I was invited into a small but vibrant circle of STS scholars, including Søren Riis, Kasper Risbjerg Eskildsen, Anders Blok, Casper Bruun Jensen, and Cathrine Hasse. My thanks for their warm companionship and inspiring intellectual engagement. My Dickinson colleagues

Wendell Smith and Marie Helweg-Larsen helped me navigate life in Copenhagen and invited me to their summer home for some needed rest and relaxation. I am grateful to Alexis Brinkemper and Olivia Heidrich for arranging my visits to Cyberdyne Care Robotics and to Yudai Katami and Kyra Hellwig for reviewing portions of the manuscript about the HAL exoskeleton.

Research for this book would not have been possible without the support of grants from the Japan Foundation, the American Council of Learned Societies (ACLS), and the Northeast Asia Council Japan Studies. While on visits to Japan, I was fortunate to be affiliated with the International Research Center for Japanese Studies in Kyoto and the Interfaculty Initiative in Information Studies at the University of Tokyo. During a year of writing on fellowship in Boston, the Reischauer Institute for Japanese Studies at Harvard University provided me with an office and intellectual home. Awards from the Dickinson Research and Development Committee helped fund research trips abroad, as well as assistance with the transcription and translation of interviews by Ibuki Aiba, Madison Alley, Miho Arai, Honoka Kawai, Catherine Lara, Shogo Nishimura, Carol Ryan, Adam Stoltenberg, and Chie Tokuyama.

Portions of chapter 3 appeared as a chapter entitled "The Work of Care in the Age of Feeling Machines" in Micky Lee and Peichi Chung, eds., *Media Technologies for Work and Play in East Asia* (Bristol: Bristol University Press, 2021) and are used here with permission.

My editor at Stanford University Press, Dylan Kyung-lim White, has been enthusiastic about and supportive of this project since we first had the opportunity to discuss it. I thank him for his expert guidance through the review process and Austin Michael Araujo for his assistance with the logistics of manuscript preparation. The book would not read as cleanly and precisely without the expert copyedits of Paul Tyler. I am grateful for his careful attention and for Tere Mullin's thoughtful construction of the book's index.

Writing is a solitary task. Books develop in conversation with many others, but they only become books through work alone in offices or, preferably in my case, among others in coffee shops and in libraries. The support of my parents, brother, and sister helped me navigate rough spots in my research and writing, and I thank them for their unconditional love and generosity. My wife, Elizabeth, has been an unyielding source of encouragement and support through the many ebbs and flows of this project. I cannot thank her enough for sacrifices of time she made on my behalf and for the many hours she listened patiently as I talked about my work (perhaps a bit too much). I dedicate this book to her and to my daughter, Noa, who reminds me every day what is wondrous about life and inspires in me boundless hope for the future.

NOTES

Preface

1. For the Fifth Science and Technology Basic Plan, see http://www.mext.go.jp
/en/policy/science_technology/lawandplan/title01/detail01/1375311.htm. For the
Cabinet Office website for Society 5.0, see https://www8.cao.go.jp/cstp/english/
society5_0/index.html.

2. Most scholarship to date focuses on the transformation of feedback relations
into digital data, particularly the troubling ways in which the algorithmic processing of digital "big data" affects constructions of self and other, provides new means
of extracting value, and reinscribes relations of inequality (Benjamin 2019; Besteman and Gusterson 2019; Boellstorff and Maurer 2015; Cheney-Lippold 2017; Eubanks 2019; Lupton 2013; Nafus 2017; Noble 2018; Rosenblat 2018; Ruckenstein and
Schüll 2017; Zuboff 2020). This book instead reorients analysis away from the products of iterative engagement—who we are through digital data—and toward *processes* of iterative engagement—who we become in everyday interaction with digital
devices that are transformed in response to their interactions with us.

Introduction

1. In this book, I use pseudonyms to refer to all individuals who are not public
figures.

2. For mass-market writing in English on robots and related digital technologies like AI, see Brynjolfsson and McAfee 2014; Ford 2015; Hornyak 2006; Markoff 2015; McAfee and Brynjolfsson 2017; White 2015. On the "robotic moment," see Turkle 2011.

3. In 1989, the total fertility rate dropped to 1.53. Fertility rates had been dropping for some time, but in this year rates fell below an aberrantly low rate in 1966.

4. This work has continued since I started my study. It is a multidisciplinary and voluminous literature, so I restrict my references here to work in Japan or with the robots that are the subject of this study. James Wright's research (Wright 2023) in a nursing home that trialed different kinds of care robots is exceptional in its level of ethnographic detail and its insight into the work of care robots within institutional settings. Yet it sheds little light on how staff and patients view care robots beyond experimental trials. Neven and Leeson (2015) include a brief description and analysis of how Paro is used in one Japanese nursing home, although it is unclear whether this was part of a regular therapeutic program or field test. The STS scholar Selma Šabanović has explored the responses of elderly individuals to Paro in the United States in field studies with colleagues (see, for example, Šabanović et al. 2013; Šabanović and Chang 2016) and in collaboration with Takanori Shibata, the inventor of Paro (Shibata et al. 2009). Dr. Shibata and his collaborators have also lab-tested and field-tested Paro in Japan over varying lengths of time (Shibata 2012; Wada et al. 2005a, 2005b, 2005c; Wada and Shibata 2007, 2008; Wada, Shibata, and Kawaguchi 2009). The anthropologist Sherry Turkle (2011) includes reports from short-term field studies with Paro in nursing homes in the United States. Scholars have also examined Paro in eldercare in Norway, Denmark, the UK, Germany, Australia, and New Zealand (Hansen, Andersen, and Bak 2010; Jøranson et al. 2016; Klein, Gaedt, and Cook 2013; Moyle et al. 2012; Robinson et al. 2013). The work on Paro in German nursing homes by the sociologists Pfadenhauer and Dukat (2015) is atypical in that it *does* focus, like mine, on institutions where Paro has been integrated into everyday care. I am not aware of field studies on the use of HAL in care, aside from those conducted by Prof. Sankai and his associates. I also do not know of any studies of AIBO in care, except for research published by members of the group in Japan whom I studied. Akinori Kubo (2013) examines how AIBO users interact with their robots but does not engage practices of care.

5. Iterative development is also called "agile development." The principles of quick deployment and rapid redevelopment in response to feedback are common to both. See Sommerville 2016, 72–100.

6. These versions are, to use Bialski's pithy phrase, "good enough" (Bialski 2024).

7. In 2014, the company changed this motto to "move fast with stable infra" (Murphy 2014).

8. The ancient Chinese sexagenary cycle assigns one of five elements and one of twelve animals to each year. According to this cycle, 1966 was a Year of the Fire

Horse *(hinoeuma)*. Superstition holds that girls born in a Fire Horse year have difficult personalities and will drive their husbands to an early death. There were 400,000 fewer births this year than in 1965, a sudden drop that many attribute to the influence of this belief.

9. See Young 1998; Norgren 2001.

10. This legislation bore the influence of global eugenics discourse and attempted to engender a larger but higher "quality" population. See Miyake 1991; Robertson 2002.

11. Numerous scholars have described the trend toward the socialization of care in Japan. For an overview, see Thang 2011.

12. See JARA and JMF (2001); Yokoyama (2004). These forecasts were significantly revised in later Ministry of Health, Labor, and Welfare (MHLW) documents, raising the projected value of industrial markets and lowering those for nonindustrial applications (Wagner 2010). For a critique of earlier projections, see Arai 2009.

13. As Armstrong et al. also note, "Major advances made in diagnostic technologies . . . seemed to offer a more 'objective' approach to diagnosis than . . . symptom reporting" (Armstrong et al. 2007, 581). Blood tests, MRI scans, biopsies, and genetic tests offered more reliable and precise methods for determining the nature of underlying pathology or presence of presymptomatic or asymptomatic biomarkers than patient interviews.

14. See Clarke et al. 2003; Lupton 2013; Nafus 2017; Ruckenstein and Schüll 2017.

15. Most of these studies have appeared since 2010, not coincidentally the year when iPhone and Android phones went mainstream (Stern 2019). On surveillance, big data, and algorithms, see Benjamin 2019; boyd and Crawford 2012; Cheney-Lippold 2017; Eubanks 2019; Lowrie 2018; Rosenblat 2018; Seaver 2022; Wilf 2013; Zuboff 2020. On digital labor, see Gray and Suri 2019; Irani 2015; Lukács 2020; Marwick 2014. On the psychological impact of smartphones and social media, see boyd 2014; Twenge 2017; Turkle 2011.

16. Perhaps more than in other languages, "robot" *(robotto)* has a conceptual promiscuity in Japanese. The term can refer to an autonomous machine, as it can to technologies that are robotic. In addition, the term connotes cutting-edge in a way that lends a certain cachet to the object in question, like the terms "smart" and "digital" do in English. This elision helps make clear why the Japanese category of "robot" can include devices as distinct as AIBO robot dogs and HAL exoskeletons.

17. Although this book is not about smartphones, the fact that it was researched and written in the era of rising smartphone adoption around the world resonates through its pages. From the debut of the iPhone in 2007 until 2020, global shipments of the device grew by double-digit percentages every year. The same is true for all classes of smartphones until 2015. Global sales of smartphones have hovered around 1.5 billion globally each year since then (Swearingen 2018; statista.com

2020). Ironically, despite the country's formative role in creating the platforms and business models on which all smartphones run, this same period saw Japanese influence on mobile phone communications recede (Steinberg 2019, 174–75).

Chapter One

1. RoboCity CoRE was slated to open in 2011 but continued to be delayed until it was ultimately abandoned. Corporate supporters of the project left when a new municipal government led by the conservative mayor Hashimoto Tōru revoked the tax breaks that they had been promised. Prof. Sano suggested to me that the mayor's decision was meant as a performative demonstration of authority over the prefectural governor regarding who ought to control regional development and planning.

2. In making this argument, I draw on a growing body of scholarship in anthropology and sociology on the role of risk in modern society. While some scholars focus on the risk of harm as a condition of late modernity (Beck 1992; Giddens 1990), others conceive of risk assessment as a calculative technology that helps manage future uncertainty, whether the risk is of something bad happening or of something good happening. Managing uncertainty through risk can generate value, for example, in financial markets, or built environments, such as antiterrorism infrastructure (Arnoldi 2004; Dean 1998; Lakoff 2008; Samimian-Darash 2011, 2013; Zaloom 2004). In this way, "risks," as the German sociologist Ulrich Beck writes, "are a kind of *virtual*, yet *real*, reality" (Beck 1998, 11, my emphasis). The expectation of a possible future can affect behavior in the present by means of its *virtual* presence. By guiding action in the present, an imagined future comes to be enacted *in practice*. Developing robotics for the future of aging, I argue, helps make its virtual presence palpable in the present.

3. One frequently heard criticism about Japan's enthusiasm for robotics is that the country prefers technological solutions over those that rely on the labor of immigrants. I put this question to a representative from one of the firms involved in the warehouse demonstration. While his parent company already employs immigrant workers in its factories, he told me that it is much harder to hire immigrant workers as delivery workers. These jobs are typically performed by one worker alone. Very few recent immigrants have the language skills and knowledge of local geography in order to carry out the work alone. However, he stressed that he looked forward to a day when more qualified foreign workers were available to fill the job needs of companies like his. His nuanced response suggests that a preference for technological solutions can stem from the demands of a particular kind of job rather than nativist impulses alone.

4. See European Commission 2009; United Nations 2001; World Bank 1994.

5. The anthropologist Felicity Aulino uses this term to describe the feedback loops that entangle government population forecasts and scholarly analyses of demographic change with the ways in which people imagine themselves in the present

and future, thus signaling the co-constitution of "demographic studies, (trans)national discourse, and individual narratives" (Aulino 2017, 321). For early and influential scholarly anthologies on Japan's aging society in English, see Coulmas 2007, 2008; Matanle, Rausch, and Shrinking Regions Research Group 2011; Traphagan and Knight 2003.

6. Notestein 1945; Omran 1971; Rostow 1990; Thompson 1929.

7. Still, the earliest proponents of demographic transition theory did not anticipate the emergence of so-called aging societies about a century later, perhaps influenced by their assumption of progressivism. For an insightful feminist analysis of early theorists of demography and population, see Murphy 2017.

8. For an analysis so deeply rooted in the study of utopianism and planning for the future, Scott's work is noticeably bereft of an extended discussion on the temporalities of planning. This is true also for critics of his work, who tend instead to fault his exclusive focus on state actors and failure to consider the influence of nonstate actors like global NGOs or multinational corporations (Coronil 2001; Ferguson 2005; Li 2005).

9. Sherry Turkle has mentioned as well the tendency of researchers to preface discussions of robotics innovation with PowerPoint presentations on Japan's worrisome demographic trends (Turkle 2011, 323n6).

10. This was the opinion as of 2011. In 2013, the Japanese government began finalizing funding for an advanced technology research center, modeled after DARPA (some have dubbed it JARPA), which would "tap a broad swath of civilian technologies with potential military uses" (Kelly and Takenaka 2013). While regional security is likely at the center of interest in funding such a facility, it is also possible that the failure to prepare adequately for the harsh conditions at Fukushima played a role as well.

11. *Japan Times* 2011; Kawatsuma, Fukushima, and Okada 2012; Onishi 2011; Penney 2012.

12. AIST is based in Tsukuba and also incubated early work on Paro and HAL. See the IRID website at https://irid.or.jp/en/.

13. https://fukushima.jaea.go.jp/en/pamphlet/pdf/naraha.pdf.

14. Ryo Morimoto, personal communication, November 30, 2023.

Chapter Two

1. On Robot Town Kyushu, see Hasegawa 2008; Hasegawa et al. 2007; Kurazume et al. 2008. On the Gifu projects, see Inaba and Chihara 2004. On Robot Town Tsukuba, see https://www.rt-tsukuba.jp.

2. CoRE is an acronym for "Center of Robotics Experiments." The association of CoRE with the English word "core" is intentional.

3. Prof. Sano thought this term was confusing in both Japanese and English. The planners intend it to mean something like "intellectual capital."

4. RoboCity appears similar to what might be known today as a "smart city."

Yet references to "smart" are entirely absent from the literature related to the project and did not emerge in any conversation with those involved in it. Conceptually, too, imagining the city as an organism that can feel, think, and act departs from the disembodied Cartesianism of smart cities. Perhaps more surprising is the lack of reference to the midcentury Japanese Metabolist movement, where understandings of biological processes were applied to architectural problems and urban design. This is especially the case given the proximity of Osaka University to the site of Expo 1970, which was in part constructed on Metabolist design principles.

5. The project was initially called the Project for the Popularization and Promotion of Robots for the Fields of Nursing Care and Medicine *(kaigo-iryō bunya robotto fukyū suishin jigyō)*.

6. Two additional technologies included in the project were NemuriSCAN, a panel that lies under a mattress and indicates if a person is in bed or not, and Readable, a machine that helps a person with limited use of the hands read printed materials.

7. At the time, LTCI reduced the cost of medical or care devices by 90 percent.

8. As I discuss in chapter 5, this contrasts with the use of HAL in Germany where the treatment of traumatic spinal cord injuries predominates.

9. The following year, in 2015, HAL was approved for manufacture and sale as a medical device in Japan.

10. I was not granted permission to observe training sessions with HAL at the RoboCare Center. However, I did have the opportunity to observe HAL therapy in Germany, where many of the same principles apply (see chapter 5).

11. The prefecture recently announced a third phase set to run through 2027 with the twin aims of facilitating the entry of small and medium-sized companies into the robot industry and encouraging the adoption of robotics technology in institutions where they might prove helpful.

12. https://sagamirobot.pref.kanagawa.jp/img/important_project/project_list/r01-report.pdf.

Chapter Three

1. *New York Times*, "133 Japanese on Airliner Die as It Crashes into Tokyo Bay," February 5, 1966.

2. *Time Magazine*, "The Worst Single Day," March 11, 1966, p. 33.

3. In Bender (2021), I explore how this shift in focus is also shaded by contemporaneous alarm about escalating rates of "lonely death" *(kodokushi)* among the elderly and of fraying social ties in Japan more generally (see also Allison 2015; Nozawa 2015).

4. For a detailed analysis of these related terms, see Roquet 2009.

5. In subsequent years, the group would adjust this somewhat cumbersome naming and go by Robot Therapy Group *(robot serapii bukai)* alone. The naming

elides the element of robotic assistance that is present in the original, but the notion of robots as assistants nevertheless remains in therapy sessions.

6. The technical term for this engineering design is "subsumption architecture" (see Kubo 2013).

7. Here I am more interested in *how* the students conducted their experiments, rather than the results of the experiment itself. They did present the results of their intervention at a meeting of the group later in the year. Their preliminary findings were that the controlled interaction with the robot slightly decreased the expression of her symptoms.

8. The "phatic function" of language is one of linguist Roman Jakobson's six functions of language (Jakobson 1990). Jakobson developed this notion from earlier work by the anthropologist Bronislaw Malinowski, who called the social ties created through regular but not necessarily meaningful exchange "phatic communion" (see Malinowski 1936). Anthropologists have examined the infrastructural dimensions of phatic communication (Elyachar 2010; Kockelman 2010) and have noted how the absence of phaticity can signal social disconnection (Nozawa 2015).

9. Level of LTCI support *(yōkaigodo)*, indexes of mobility *(netakirido)*, and dementia severity *(ninchishōdo)* are determined by care managers at the municipal office together with medical professionals. They are indexed on scales ascending from 1 to 5, A1 to C2, and I through IV, respectively.

10. There is extensive scholarship on the roles that women play in caring for children and the elderly in Japan, both in households and in institutional settings. See, for example, Allison 2000; Jenike 2003; Traphagen 2006; White 2002.

11. The group uses the diminutive honorific *"-chan"* to refer to the robot dog in the same way that one might refer to a pet animal. The group never suggested that the animaloid robots that they used were living animals when asked by residents. Both residents and group members would nevertheless use honorifics like *"-chan"* when referring to robots in the midst of a session. Even though all were aware that the robots were not alive, the use of this honorific practically elides the distinctions of organic being and inorganic machine in the linguistic flow of therapy sessions. The group's remote control of AIBO in particular enhanced, either intentionally or unintentionally, this blurring of conceptual boundaries.

Chapter Four

1. https://worldhappiness.report/.

2. In a 2011 interview, I asked one of Paro's developers about the Guinness World Record. References to the award frequently appear in advertisements for Paro and are often mentioned in scholarship about it. The developer told me that it seemed to him like a publicity stunt. The designation originated in a chance encounter between editors of the Guinness Book and the makers of Paro in London in 2002. During that time, Paro was displayed alongside Sony's AIBO and other

gadgets from Japan at an exhibition at the Science Museum in London called "Japan: Gateway to the Future." The editors visited the exhibit and were intrigued by Paro. They told the makers of device that they were interested in including it in their book and asked if there was any scientific data available related to its use. "So, we sent them a recent article and they created a new category of robot called 'Therapy Robot,' and designated Paro as the Most Therapeutic Robot in the world. Of course, at the time, there were really no other 'therapy robots' in existence. It'd be hard to compare differences in therapeutic effect, even if there were" (interview, June 2011). As the basis of the award derives from one of many experiments with the device, it's not clear that it would be as well advertised had Paro not been taken up later in dementia care in Denmark.

3. Denmark's Council on Ethics routinely reviews new products intended for healthcare among other purposes (https://www.etiskraad.dk/english).

4. Some roboticists I met in Japan suggested that the decision to model Paro on a seal helped to solve engineering challenges. It's much more difficult to engineer the movements of a robot dog or cat. Fine motor control of multiple limbs on an autonomous, mobile machine is a significant technical hurdle.

5. The emphasis on addressing the subjective needs and wants of individuals links PCC with other forms of patient-centered care in clinical medicine (Armstrong 1984; Sullivan 2003).

6. This usage is awkward in English writing outside this specific context. For this reason, I instead use the term "residents" in this chapter.

7. When talking with me in English, Danish care workers would often flip the word and say "life quality," which retains the order of the Danish root words that make up the term for quality of life, *livskvalitet*.

8. The ethics of using Paro are also covered at the certification workshop, so it is not surprising that it is on the minds of these care workers. The workshop explicitly instructs care workers to be honest about what Paro is. Family members would raise the question as well; that is, whether it was right to have older adults with dementia "play with robots." The National Ethics Council's report on Paro also considered this very issue. As a consequence, many Danish care workers had thought about it, which might account for some of the uniformity in the responses. Being truthful about Paro's status as a machine was also the typical practice in Japan.

9. Most of these have been efforts to legitimate Paro as a therapeutic device by Dr. Shibata and colleagues. See Jøranson et al. 2016; Saito et al. 2002; Shibata and Wada 2011; Shibata 2012; Wada and Shibata 2007; Wada et al. 2005a, 2005b, 2005c.

10. The title of the Japanese version is *robotto serapii no tebiki: azarashi-gata robotto "paro" no katsuyō-hō*. The Japanese version is two pages longer than the English version (32 to 30). Otherwise, the two are identical. The English is a direct translation of the original Japanese and there is no consideration of cultural difference in the application of the device.

11. Five more research conferences have been held in Japan since 2012. The most recent took place on November 1, 2018. Conferences are only open to registered users of Paro in Japan.

12. Some prefectures do offer discounts on the purchase of Paro in connection with local efforts to promote care technologies.

Chapter Five

1. In marketing materials, HAL is typically preceded by the words "robot suit." Cyberdyne calls the exoskeleton in use at CCR "robot suit HAL lower-body type."

2. Patients and therapists in Germany did not refer to the HAL suit as an exoskeleton. Instead, they called it "robot" or "robot suit." Although thinking of HAL as a robot might imply that the machine moves a person unidirectionally, German interlocutors pointed out that the HAL system *works with* a person to generate intended movement. This distinction was believed by them to be crucial in distinguishing HAL from other kinds of exoskeleton technology.

3. In Japanese-language writing on HAL, Sankai and his collaborators often use the compound word *iryō fukushi* to cover medical applications and (nonmedical) welfare applications of HAL technology with one term. This usage is not uncommon in Japanese but it can be confusing in English, which is why I treat them separately.

4. In these early descriptions, older adults and persons with disabilities are collapsed together as the kinds of individuals who would regain independence with HAL technology. In 2003, for example, the English-language *Taipei Times* newspaper described HAL as a Japanese "robot suit that helps aged or physically disabled people walk, get up the stairs or seat themselves to relax without a chair" (*Taipei Times* 2003). They are similarly conflated as the target market for the HAL device in other English-language media (Nakamura 2004; *Health Futures Digest* 2004) and in papers by Prof. Sankai and his colleagues as late as 2007 (Kawamoto and Sankai 2005; Suzuki et al. 2007).

5. A 2015 government *White Paper on Science and Technology*, for example, attributes the rationale for supporting HAL's development to "[Japan's] rapidly aging society" (MEXT 2015). A 2017 pamphlet advertising the activities of Dr. Sankai's laboratory at the University of Tsukuba similarly positions the technology as a potential answer to the "problems facing [Japan's] society like low-fertility and aging" (University of Tsukuba 2017).

6. Prof. Sankai's Cybernics is conceptually indebted to the interdisciplinary field of cybernetics, which ascended in the decades following World War II. Early cyberneticians were fascinated by the way in which biological organisms and mechanical systems can both maintain a steady state, or "homeostasis." They argued that machines and living beings maintain homeostasis through relations of feedback and response (Hayles 1999; Wiener 1948, 1950). What organisms achieve with nerves, brains, and muscles, homeostatic machines accomplish with networks of

sensors, processors, and actuators. Joining together human and machine results from the linkage of heterogeneous systems in loops of feedback. More than any other field of study, feedback is foundational to cybernetics, specifically "negative feedback"—the modification of a functioning system in response to deviation from a predetermined baseline. Nineteenth-century scientists studying electric circuits formulated understandings of feedback before the emergence of cybernetics (Mindell 2002). But, as Peter Galison has written, it was the founder of cybernetics, the mathematician Norbert Wiener, who "put feedback in the foreground" (Galison 1994, 258). In midcentury, researchers put cybernetic principles into action through experimental combinations of organisms and machines (Clynes and Kline 1960; Haraway 1997). With HAL technology, Prof. Sankai has pushed the human–machine assemblage even further.

In 2017, I asked Prof. Sankai in an interview how he distinguishes cybernics from cybernetics. He dismissed the latter as "just math." "What works in theory," he continued, "often fails in practice." He needed more than mathematical theory alone to integrate physiological systems with mechanical and information systems, which led him to found a new interdisciplinary field. Cybernics nevertheless inherits from cybernetics the view that bodies and machines are systems that self-regulate through sensing, feedback, and response.

7. In one article, for example, German researchers write: "The results of our case show plastic changes in the brain that accompany improvement. They suggest that cortical plastic changes due to improved use of the remaining intact spinal connections, rather than regeneration of the lesioned spinal connections, *might be responsible* for the functional improvement in our patients" (Sczesny-Kaiser et al. 2014: 15, my emphasis).

8. See https://www.bg-kliniken.de/en/facilities/bg-hospital-bergmannsheil-bochum/.

9. On this and a previous visit in 2015, therapy with the suit was not covered by the German health insurance system. Patients either paid out of pocket, were supported by a research study, or were covered by BG insurance. The lack of coverage for their care was a substantial obstacle for the recruitment of patients, most of whom would struggle to pay the equivalent of $500 for a two-hour training session.

10. Being tracked through digital technologies is by now a familiar experience. Smartphones, smart watches, and other wearable technologies in everyday use provide a service of value to consumers while also servicing valuable information about consumer behavior to corporations. The HAL exoskeleton demonstrates not just the expansion of robotics technology into this realm but the enrollment of sites of care into processes of technological innovation.

In a prescient 2000 article, the sociologists Kevin Haggerty and Richard Ericson write: "The concept of 'surplus value' has traditionally been associated with Marxism. For Marx, it designated how the owners of the means of production profit from workers' excess labour power for which they are not financially compensated . . . Today, however, surplus value has escaped from a purely labour-oriented discourse and can now also be located in the language of cybernetics. In a cybernetic world, surplus value increasingly refers to the profit that can be derived from *the surplus information that different populations trail behind them in their daily lives*" (Haggerty and Ericson 2000: 616–17, my emphasis). Haggerty and Ericson were writing when internet-enabled technologies of tracking were still in their infancy. Yet they recognized early on how these technologies could transform digitally mediated interactions into acts of value. Such transformations have only intensified in recent years as more and more activities in daily life are mediated by internet-connected technologies.

Terms developed by other scholars, such as "digital persona" (Clarke 1994), "digital individual" (Agre 1994), and "digital shadow" (Kilger 1994), similarly describe the construction of individual subjectivities out of surplus information. In the current age of big data, social media, and artificial intelligence, it is more common to talk about "data exhaust"—the digital effluence generated by billions of interactions mediated by the internet each day—and its commodification through aggregation and algorithmic processing (Cheney-Lippold 2017; Zuboff 2020). The data produced by patient–HAL sessions is not on the scale of the billions of data points aggregated by companies like Facebook and Google. Yet it is clearly *surplus* information generated through acts of care. What matters, it seems to me, is not the amount of data at issue but the manner in which it is produced and the way in which it is collected.

11. Freud 2003. For a provocative analysis of the robots and the uncanny, see Wilf 2019.

Chapter Six

1. In this respect, Sasuke is similar in conception to RI-MAN and RIBA, two earlier robot prototypes developed by the Japanese research institute RIKEN-HRI (Salton 2009). RI-MAN and RIBA functioned similarly to Sasuke but looked like living things—humanoid and animaloid, respectively. Neither was commercialized.

2. https://www.fuji.co.jp/en/about/hug/.

3. Based on feedback from institutional customers, the company recently released a new version of Hug that is small enough for it to be usable in domestic settings. This new model won a robot award from METI in 2021 (https://www.robotaward.jp/winning/index.html#R03).

4. As of 2022, Daiwa House no longer handles Cyberdyne's robotics products.

5. Cyberdyne simultaneously developed an iteration of HAL Lumbar Type for use by warehouse workers and manual laborers in fields other than care (HAL Lumbar Type for Labor Support). Later, they released a version for "welfare" *(fukushi)* purposes that is meant to help able-bodied people maintain or improve functional health. This is similar to the way in which the lower-body exoskeleton is

used at HAL Fit locations, but the lighter-weight lumbar-support robot requires less assistance to put on.

6. I am indebted to Søren Riis for getting me to think more about things.

7. https://robotcare.jp/data/etc/ROBOT-CARE-pamphlet_eng.pdf.

8. These are the Ministry of Education, Culture, Sports, Science, and Technology (MEXT), the Ministry of Health, Labor, and Welfare (MHLW), and Ministry of Economy, Trade, and Industry (METI). See https://www.kantei.go.jp/jp/singi/kenkouiryou/en/pdf/doc1.pdf.

9. These priority areas were expanded in 2017.

10. The standard is called the International Classification of Functioning, Disability, and Health, or ICF. See https://www.who.int/standards/classifications/international-classification-of-functioning-disability-and-health

11. https://www.dbj.jp/pdf/investigate/mo_report/0000015497_file4.pdf.

12. Communication robots are defined loosely as "assistive devices that apply robotics technology in the service of communicating with an older adult" (https://robotcare.jp/jp/priority/priority11).

13. A recent ethnographic study on trials of these new robots suggests that this may not be the case (see Wright 2023).

14. I include NemuriScan within care robotics 2.0 as another example of machines that monitor the bodies of older adults, but this particular machine has a long history of development. It was included in the same 2010 project in Kanagawa Prefecture that tested the effectiveness of Paro and the HAL lower-body exoskeleton. However, at the time, the latter two robotic devices figured much more prominently as examples of cutting-edge technologies for eldercare in Japan.

15. The Robot Therapy Group did trial a prototype of a communication robot like Palro. That prototype looked like a bear cub and had the ability to hear and to issue verbal commands through a speaker. However, unlike Palro, it could not move its limbs. The prototype was never commercialized.

16. Government of Japan 2016.

17. Government of Japan 2016, 13; https://www8.cao.go.jp/cstp/english/society5_0/.

18. See https://www8.cao.go.jp/cstp/english/society5_0/; Keidanren 2018, 4–5.

19. https://www8.cao.go.jp/cstp/english/society5_0/.

20. This unidirectionality was corrected in a report on a program grant prepared by Prof. Sankai for a government ministry. The same image appears of Cyberdyne technologies in a cartoon village. However, layered on top of this version of the image are huge bold arrows that illustrate the cyclical flow of data between Cyberdyne interfaces and the village. This addition may signal recognition after the fact of the unidirectionally extractive operation implied by the original panel image. See https://www8.cao.go.jp/cstp/sentan/kakushintekikenkyu/siryo/report5_sankai.pdf.

Epilogue

    1. https://www.softbank.jp/en/corp/group/sbm/news/press/2014/20140605_01/.

    2. Digital surveillance was particularly pronounced in South Korea, China, and Taiwan. Efforts to implement a digital contact-tracing app in Japan were ultimately unsuccessful (Borovoy 2022; Wright 2021).

    3. At the end of the preceding year, Softbank also sold off a controlling stake in Boston Dynamics to the Korean firm Hyundai (Inagaki and Song 2020).

    4. https://www.cyberdyne.jp/english/services/CybernicsTreatment.html.

    5. https://us.aibo.com/feature/ai.html.

REFERENCES

Adelstein, Jake, and David McNeill. 2011. "Meltdown: What Really Happened at Fukushima?" *The Atlantic*, July 2. https://www.theatlantic.com/international/archive/2011/07/meltdown-what-really-happened-fukushima/352434/.

Agre, Philip E. 1994. "Understanding the Digital Individual." *Information Society* 10(2): 73–76.

Allison, Anne. 2000. *Permitted and Prohibited Desires: Mothers, Comics, and Censorship in Japan.* Berkeley: University of California Press.

Allison, Anne. 2006. *Millennial Monsters: Japanese Toys and the Global Imagination.* Berkeley: University of California Press.

Allison, Anne. 2015. "Discounted Life: Social Time in Relationless Japan." *Boundary 2* 42(3): 129–41.

Ambo, Phie, dir. 2007. *Mechanical Love.* Icarus Films. 52 min.

Anderson, Ben. 2009. "Affective Atmospheres." *Emotion, Space and Society* 2(2): 77–81.

Arai, Hirohiko. 2009. "Robotto sangyō ni kan suru shijō chōsa-shijō yosoku no hikaku to bunseki" [Comparison and analysis of market surveys and forecasts on robot industry]. *Nihon robotto gakkai-shi* 27(3): 265–67.

Armstrong, David. 1984. "The Patient's View." *Social Science & Medicine* 18(9): 737–44.

Armstrong, David, Richard Lilford, Jane Ogden, and Simon Wessely. 2007. "Health-Related Quality of Life and the Transformation of Symptoms." *Sociology of Health & Illness* 29: 570–83.

Arnoldi, Jakob. 2004. "Derivatives: Virtual Values and Real Risks." *Theory, Culture & Society* 21(6): 23–42.

Aulino, Felicity. 2016. "Rituals of Care for the Elderly in Northern Thailand: Merit, Morality, and the Everyday of Long-Term Care." *American Ethnologist* 43: 91–102.

Aulino, Felicity. 2017. "Narrating the Future: Population Aging and the Demographic Imaginary in Thailand." *Medical Anthropology* 36(4): 319–31.

Bach, Jonathan. 2011. "Modernity and the Urban Imagination in Economic Zones." *Theory, Culture & Society* 28(5): 98–122.

Banno Takashi. 2023. "With Eyes on Mars, U.S. Scientists Test Japan-Made Robot Seal for Reducing Astronaut Stress." *Japan News*, January 8. https://japannews.yomiuri.co.jp/science-nature/technology/20230108-82592/.

Beck, Ulrich. 1992. *Risk Society: Toward a New Modernity*. London: Sage.

Beck, Ulrich. 1998. "Politics of Risk Society." In *The Politics of Risk Society*, edited by Jane Franklin, 9–22. Cambridge: Polity Press.

Bender, Shawn. 2021. "The Work of Care in the Age of Feeling Machines." In *Media Technologies for Work and Play in East Asia*, edited by Micky Lee and Peichi Chung, 265–82. Bristol: Bristol University Press.

Benjamin, Ruha. 2019. *Race after Technology: Abolitionist Tools for the New Jim Code*. Cambridge: Polity Press.

Besteman, Catherine, and Hugh Gusterson, ed. 2019. *Life by Algorithms: How Roboprocesses Are Remaking Our World*. Chicago: University of Chicago Press.

Bestor, Theodore. 2013. "Disasters, Natural and Unnatural: Reflections on March 11, 2011, and Its Aftermath." *Journal of Asian Studies* 72: 763–82.

Bialski, Paula. 2020. "Speeding Up, Slowing Down, Breaking Down: An Ethnography of Software-Driven Mobility." *Mobilities* 15(5): 740–55.

Bialski, Paula. 2024. *Middle Tech: Software Work and the Culture of Good Enough*. Princeton, NJ: Princeton University Press.

Boellstorff, Tom, and Bill Maurer. 2015. *Data, Now Bigger and Better!* Chicago: Prickly Paradigm Press.

Borovoy, Amy. 2022. "The Burdens of Self-Restraint: Social Measures and the Containment of Covid-19 in Japan." *Asia-Pacific Journal: Japan Focus*, December. https://apjjf.org/2022/19/Borovoy.html.

boyd, danah. 2014. *It's Complicated: The Social Lives of Networked Teens*. New Haven, CT: Yale University Press.

boyd, danah, and Kate Crawford. 2012. "Critical Questions for Big Data." *Information, Communication & Society* 15(5): 662–79.

Brooks, Rodney. 2002. *Flesh and Machines: How Robots Will Change Us.* 1st ed. New York: Pantheon Books.

Brynjolfsson, Erik, and Andrew McAfee. 2014. *The Second Machine Age: Work, Progress, and Prosperity in a Time of Brilliant Technologies.* New York: W.W. Norton, 2014.

Buch, Elana D. 2015. "Anthropology of Aging and Care." *Annual Review of Anthropology* 44(1): 277–93.

Cabinet Office of Japan. 2014. *Comprehensive Special Zone Policy.* English translation. http://www.kantei.go.jp/jp/singi/tiiki/sogotoc/siryou/gaiyoueng.pdf.

Cabinet Office of Japan. 2020. *Integrated Innovation Strategy 2020.* July 17. https://www8.cao.go.jp/cstp/english/strategy_2020.pdf.

Cabinet Office of Japan. 2021. *Science, Technology, and Innovation (STI) Basic Plan.* March 26. https://www8.cao.go.jp/cstp/english/sti_basic_plan.pdf.

Campbell, John. 2000. "Changing Meanings of Frail Old People and the Japanese Welfare State." In *Caring for the Elderly in Japan and the US: Practices and Policies,* edited by Susan Orpett Long, 84–99. London: Routledge.

Campbell, John, and Naoki Ikegami. 2000. "Long-Term Care Insurance Comes to Japan." *Health Affairs* 19(3): 26–39.

Čapek, Karel. 2004. *R.U.R. (Rossum's Universal Robots).* Translated by Claudia Novack. Introduction by Ivan Klíma. New York: Penguin Books.

Carse, Ashley, and David Kneas. 2019. "Unbuilt and Unfinished: The Temporalities of Infrastructure." *Environment and Society* 10(1): 9–28.

Chen, Steven. 2012. "The Rise of Sōshokukei Danshi Masculinity and Consumption in Contemporary Japan: A Historic and Discursive Analysis." In *Gender, Culture, and Consumer Behavior,* edited by Cele Otnes and Linda Zayer, 285–310. New York: Routledge.

Cheney-Lippold, John. 2017. *We Are Data: Algorithms and the Making of Our Digital Selves.* New York: New York University Press.

Chino Keiko and Yoshida Noriyuki. 2011. "Tsukaenai nihonsei robotto, genpatsu saigai ni nōryoku busoku (kaisetsu)" [Useless Japanese robots: Failure to respond to nuclear disaster]. *Yomiuri Shinbun,* morning ed., April 20, p. 11.

Clarke, Adele E., Janet K. Shim, Laura Mamo, Jennifer Ruth Fosket, and Jennifer R. Fishman. 2003. "Biomedicalization: Technoscientific Transformations of Health, Illness, and U.S. Biomedicine." *American Sociological Review* 68(2): 161–94.

Clarke, Roger. 1994. "The Digital Persona and Its Application to Data Surveillance." *Information Society* 10(2): 77–92.

Clynes, Manfred E., and Nathan S. Kline. 1960. "Cyborgs and Space." *Astronautics* 5(9): 26–27, 74–76.

Coronil, Fernando. 2001. "Smelling Like a Market." *American Historical Review* 106(1): 119–29.

Coulmas, Florian. 2007. *Population Decline and Ageing in Japan: The Social Consequences*. London: Routledge.

Coulmas, Florian, ed. 2008. *The Demographic Challenge: A Handbook about Japan*. Boston: Brill.

Cross, Jamie. 2015. "The Economy of Anticipation." *Comparative Studies of South Asia Africa and the Middle East* 35(3): 424–37.

Cruciger, Oliver, Thomas A. Schildhauer, Renate C. Meindl, Martin Tegenthoff, Peter Schwenkreis, Mustafa Citak, and Mirko Aach. 2016. "Impact of Locomotion Training with a Neurologic Controlled Hybrid Assistive Limb (HAL) Exoskeleton on Neuropathic Pain and Health-Related Quality of Life (HRQoL) in Chronic SCI: A Case Study." *Disability & Rehabilitation: Assistive Technology* 11(6): 529–34.

Dahler, Anne Marie. 2018. "Welfare Technologies and Ageing Bodies: Various Ways of Practising Autonomy." *Hindawi: Rehabilitation Research and Practice*, pp. 1–9.

Daiwa House Corp. n.d. "Hisaichi no shisetsu ni hirogaru egao no wa" [Bringing smiles to faces in disaster shelters]. Press release. https://www.daiwahouse.co.jp /robot/paro/case/case01.html.

Davies, Alex. 2019. "This Food-Delivery Robot Wants to Share the Bike Lane." *Wired*. https://www.wired.com/story/food-delivery-robot-wants-share-bike-lane/.

Dean, Mitchell. 1998. "Risk: Calculable and Incalculable." *Soziale Welt: Zeitschrift für sozialwissenschaftliche Forschung und Praxis* 49: 25–42.

Deguchi, Atsushi, Chiaki Hirai, Hideyuki Matsuoka, Taku Nakano, Kohei Oshima, Mitsuharu Tai, and Shigeyuki Tani. 2020. "What Is Society 5.0?" In *Society 5.0*, edited by Hitachi-UTokyo Laboratory, 1–23. Singapore: Springer.

Digital Agency (Japan). 2021. *Outline of the Basic Act on the Formation of a Digital Society*. September 1. https://www.digital.go.jp/assets/contents/node/basic_ page/field_ref_resources/0f321c23-517f-439e-9076-5804f0a24b59/20210901_en_ 01.pdf.

Dumit, Joseph. 2012. *Drugs for Life: How Pharmaceutical Companies Define Our Health*. Durham, NC: Duke University Press.

Dyer-Witheford, Nick. 2015. *Cyber-Proletariat: Global Labour in the Digital Vortex*. London: Pluto Press.

Elyachar, Julia. 2010. "Phatic Labor, Infrastructure, and the Question of Empowerment in Cairo." *American Ethnologist* 37(3): 452–64.

Engelberger, Joseph F. 1985. "The Ultimate Worker." In *Robotics*, edited by Marvin Minsky, 184–213. New York: Anchor Press/Doubleday.

Estes, Adam Clarke. 2011. "Japan Invents a Cyborg Suit to Clean Up Fukushima." *The Atlantic*, November 8. https://www.theatlantic.com/technology/archive/ 2011/11/japan-invents-cyborg-suit-clean-fukushima/335769/.

Eubanks, Virginia. 2019. *Automating Inequality: How High-Tech Tools Profile, Police, and Punish the Poor*. New York: St. Martin's Press.

European Commission. 2009. *Ageing Report: Economic and Budgetary Projections for the EU-27 Member States (2008–2060)*. Brussels: European Communities. http://www.da.dk/bilag/publication14992_ageing_report.pdf.

Ferguson, James. 2005. "Seeing Like an Oil Company: Space, Security, and Global Capital in Neoliberal Africa." *American Anthropologist* 107: 377–82.

Fisch, Michael. 2019. *An Anthropology of the Machine: Tokyo's Commuter Train Network*. Chicago: University of Chicago Press.

Fisch, Michael. n.d. "Meditations on the 'Unimaginable' *(sōteigai)*." In *The Space of Disaster*, edited by Erez Golani Solomon. Tel-Aviv: Resling.

Ford, Martin. 2015. *Rise of the Robots: Technology and the Threat of a Jobless Future*. New York: Basic Books.

Freud, Sigmund. 2003. *The Uncanny*. Translated by David McLintock, with an introduction by Hugh Haughton. New York: Penguin Books.

Frumer, Yulia. 2018a. "Beyond Singular Tasks: Labor-Saving Technologies and Systems of Labor." In *Expert Voices on Japan Security, Economic, Social, and Foreign Policy Recommendations: U.S.-Japan Network for the Future Cohort IV*, edited by Arthur Alexander, 33–47. Washington, DC: Maureen and Mike Mansfield Foundation.

Frumer, Yulia. 2018b. "Cognition and Emotions in Japanese Humanoid Robotics." *History and Technology* 34(2): 157–83.

Fujita, Masahiro. 2001. "AIBO: Toward the Era of Digital Creatures." *The International Journal of Robotics Research* 20(10): 781–794.

Fujita, Masahiro. 2004. "On Activating Human Communications with Pet-Type Robot AIBO." *Proceedings of the IEEE* 92(11): 1804–13.

Galbraith, Patrick W. 2019. *Otaku and the Struggle for Imagination in Japan*. Durham, NC: Duke University Press.

Galison, Peter. 1994. "The Ontology of the Enemy: Norbert Wiener and the Cybernetic Vision." *Critical Inquiry* 21: 228–66.

Giddens, Anthony. 1990. *The Consequences of Modernity*. Stanford, CA: Stanford University Press.

Gjødsbøl, Iben, Lene Koch, and Mette N. Svendsen. 2017. "Resisting Decay: On Disposal, Valuation, and Care in a Dementia Nursing Home in Denmark." *Social Science & Medicine* 184: 116–23.

Good Tree, Corp. n.d. "Kea no ki de hakaru" [Health tracking with care devices]. Unpublished pamphlet.

Government of Japan. 2016. *Report on the 5th Science and Technology Basic Plan*. Provisional translation, January 22.

Gray, Mary, and Siddharth Suri. 2019. *Ghost Work: How to Stop Silicon Valley from Building a New Global Underclass*. New York: Houghton Mifflin Harcourt.

Guinness World Records. 2003. "Most Therapeutic Robot." Bantam: London, p. 167.

Haggerty, Kevin D., and Richard V. Ericson. 2000. "The Surveillant Assemblage." *British Journal of Sociology* 51: 605–22.

Hansen, Søren Tranberg, Hans Jorgen Andersen, and Thomas Bak. 2010. "Practical Evaluation of Robots for Elderly in Denmark—An Overview." *Proceedings of the 5th ACM/IEEE International Conference on Human-Robot Interaction*, Osaka, pp. 149–50.

Haraway, Donna. 1997. *Modest_Witness@Second_Millennium.FemaleMan_Meets_OncoMouse: Feminism and Technoscience*. New York: Routledge.

Hasegawa Tsutomu. 2008. "Kankyō purattofōmu 'robot taun'" [Robot Town: A robotics structured environment platform]. *Journal of the Robotics Society of Japan* 26(5): 411–14.

Hasegawa Tsutomu, Ryo Kurazume, Kouji Murakami, Yoshihiko Kimuro, Takashi Ienaga, Daisaku Arita, Yōsuke Senda, Masaru Adachi, Kazuhiko Yokoyama. 2007. *Robot Town Project*. http://rraj.rsj-web.org/en_atcl/945%5B12/31/17.

Hayles, N. Katherine. 1999. *How We Became Posthuman: Virtual Bodies in Cybernetics, Literature, and Informatics*. Chicago: University of Chicago Press.

Health Futures Digest. 2004. "Another Exoskeleton for the Closet." September, p. 66.

Hetherington, Kregg. 2016. "Surveying the Future Perfect: Anthropology, Development and the Promise of Infrastructure." In *Infrastructures and Social Complexity: A Routledge Companion*, edited by Penny Harvey, Casper Bruun Jensen and Atsuro Morita, 40–50. London: Routledge.

Hornyak, Timothy N. 2006. *Loving the Machine: The Art and Science of Japanese Robots*. Tokyo: Kodansha International.

Hornyak, Tim. 2007. "Robotopia Rising: Next Generation of Robots in Japan Brings SF Closer to Fact." *Japan Spotlight*, January/February.

Inaba, Akio, and Kenji Chihara. 2004. "The Gifu Robot Project 21" [Gifu robotto purojekuto 21]. *Journal of the Robotics Society of Japan* 22(7): 818–21.

Inagaki, Kana, and Song Jung-a. 2020. "SoftBank Sells Robot-Maker Boston Dynamics in $1.1bn Deal with Hyundai." *Financial Times*, December 11.

Intelligent Systems, Co. 2013. "Shin-gata serapii-yō azarashi-gata mentarukomitto-robotto paro ga tōjō" [New version of mental commitment seal robot Paro for therapeutic use released]. Press release, September 13.

Irani, Lilly. 2015. "Difference and Dependence among Digital Workers: The Case of Amazon Mechanical Turk." *South Atlantic Quarterly* 114(1): 225–34.

Jakobson, Roman. 1990. "The Speech Event and the Function of Language." In *On Language*, edited by Linda R. Waugh and Monique Monville-Burston, 69–79. Cambridge, MA: Harvard University Press.

JARA (Japan Robot Association) and JMF (Japan Machinery Federation). 2001. *Nijūisseiki ni okeru robotto shakai-sōzō no tame no gijutsu-senryaku chōsa-hōkokusho* [Report on the technology strategy for creating a "robot society" in the twenty-first century]. May.

Japan Times. 2011. "Japanese Robots Await Call to Action." April 23. www.japan times.co.jp/news/2011/04/23/news/japanese-robots-await-call-to-action/.

Jasanoff, Sheila, and Sang-Hyun Kim. 2015. *Dreamscapes of Modernity: Sociotechnical Imaginaries and the Fabrication of Power*. Chicago: University of Chicago Press.

Jenike, Brenda. 2003. "Parent Care and Shifting Family Obligations in Urban Japan." In *Demographic Change and the Family in Japan's Aging Society*, edited by John Traphagen and John Knight, 177–201. Albany: SUNY Press.

Jøranson, Nina, Ingeborg Pedersen, Anne Marie Mork Rokstad, and Camilla Ihlebæk. 2016. "Change in Quality of Life in Older People with Dementia Participating in Paro-Activity: A Cluster-Randomized Controlled Trial." *Journal of Advanced Nursing* 72(12): 3020–33.

Kajitani, Isamu, and Yujin Wakita 2017 "An Introduction to the Development of Transfer Assistive Robots in Japan." In *Harnessing the Power of Technology to Improve Lives*, edited by Peter Cudd and Luc de Witte, 465–71. Amsterdam: IOS Press.

Kanamic, Corp. n.d. "Jinsei wo Daki-shimeru kuraudo" [The cloud that embraces your life]. Unpublished pamphlet.

Katz, Sidney, Amasa Ford, Roland Moskowitz, Beverly Jackson, and Marjorie Jaffe. 1963. "Studies of Illness in the Aged–The Index of ADL: A Standardized Measure of Biological and Psychosocial Function." *Journal of the American Medical Association* 185: 914–19.

Kawamoto Hiroki and Yoshiyuki Sankai. 2005 "Power Assist Method Based on Phase Sequence and Muscle Force Condition for HAL." *Advanced Robotics* 19(7): 717–34.

Kawatsuma, Shinji, Mineo Fukushima, and Takashi Okada. 2012. "Emergency Response by Robots to Fukushima-Daiichi Accident: Summary and Lessons Learned." *Industrial Robot* 39(5): 428–35.

Keidanren (Japan Business Federation). 2018. "Society 5.0: Co-Creating the Future." https://www.keidanren.or.jp/en/policy/2018/095_booklet.pdf.

Kelly, Tim, and Kiyoshi Takenaka. 2013. "Japan to Tap Technology for Military Use, Another Step Away from Pacifism." *Reuters UK*, November 13. http://uk .reuters.com/article/2013/11/13/uk-japan-defence-idUKBRE9ACoDH20131113.

Kilger, Max. 1994. "The Digital Individual." *Information Society* 10(2): 93–99.

Kitazawa Kochi. 2015. "The Fukushima Nuclear Accident: Lost Opportunities and the 'Safety Myth.'" In *Examining Japan's Lost Decades*, edited by Yoichi Funabashi and Barak Kushner, 118–34. New York: Routledge.

Kitwood, Tom. 1997. *Dementia Reconsidered: The Person Comes First*. Philadelphia: Open University Press.

Klein, Barbara, Lone Gaedt, and Glenda Cook. 2013. "Emotional Robots: Principles and Experiences with Paro in Denmark, Germany, and the UK." *Journal of Gerontopsychology and Geriatric Psychiatry* 26(2): 89–99.

Kleinman, Arthur, and Hall-Clifford, Rachel. 2010. "Afterword: Chronicity—Time, Space, and Culture." In *Chronic Conditions, Fluid States: Chronicity and the Anthropology of Illness*, edited by Lenore Manderson and Carolyn Smith-Morris, 247–52. New Brunswick, NJ: Rutgers University Press.

KLIP (Kanagawa Prefecture Labor and Industry Promotion Division). 2012. *Chiiki kasseikai sōgō tokubetsu kuiki shitei shinseisho* [Application for designation as a comprehensive special zone]. September 28. http://www.pref.kanagawa.jp/documents/15368/474348.pdf.

KMO (Knowledge Capital Management Corporation) n.d. *Knowledge Capital.* Brochure. Osaka: KMO.

Kockelman, Paul. 2010. "Enemies, Parasites, and Noise: How to Take Up Residence in a System without Becoming a Term in It." *Journal of Linguistic Anthropology* 20(2): 406–21.

Kontos, Pia C. 2005. "Embodied Selfhood in Alzheimer's Disease: Rethinking Person-Centred Care." *Dementia* 4(4): 553–70.

Kubo Akinori. 2013. "Plastic Comparison: The Case of Engineering and Living with Pet-Type Robots in Japan." *East Asian Science, Technology and Society: An International Journal* 7(2): 205–20.

Kurazume, Ryo, Kōji Murakami, Yoshihiko Kimuro, Takafumi Ienaga, Shinichi Baba, and Zhongxiang Yin. 2008. "Robotto taun no kyōtsū purattofōmu gijutsu no mekanizumu" [Technical introduction of the common platform in Robot Town project]. *Journal of the Robotics Society of Japan* 26(5): 415–19.

Kusuda, Yoshihiro. 2006. "How Japan Sees the Robotics for the Future: Observation at the World Expo 2005." *Industrial Robot* 33(1): 11–18.

KWSA (Kanagawa Welfare Service Association). 2011. *2010-nendo kaigo iryō bunya robotto fukyū suishin jigyō saishū hōkokusho* [Report on the nursing-care robot promotion project]. Report, February 28.

Lakoff, Andrew. 2008. "The Generic Biothreat, or, How We Became Unprepared." *Cultural Anthropology* 23(3): 399–423.

Latour, Bruno, and Steve Woolgar. 1986. *Laboratory Life: The Construction of Scientific Facts.* Princeton, NJ: Princeton University Press.

Li, Tania Murray. 2005. "Beyond 'The State' and Failed Schemes." *American Anthropologist* 107(3): 383–394.

Lowrie, Ian. 2018. "Algorithms and Automation: An Introduction." *Cultural Anthropology* 33(3): 349–59.

Lukács, Gabriella. 2020. *Invisibility by Design: Women and Labor in Japan's Digital Economy.* Durham: Duke University Press.

Lupton, Deborah. 2013. "Quantifying the Body: Monitoring and Measuring Health in the Age of mHealth Technologies." *Critical Public Health* 23: 393–403.

Lupton, Deborah. 2019. *Data Selves: More-than-Human Perspectives.* Medford, MA: Polity.

Malinowski, Bronislaw. 1936. "The Problem of Meaning in Primitive Languages." In *The Meaning of Meaning*, edited by Charles K. Ogden and Ian A. Richards, 296–336. New York: Harcourt, Brace.

Markoff, John. 2015. *Machines of Loving Grace: The Quest for Common Ground between Humans and Robots*. New York: Ecco.

Marwick, Alice. 2014. *Status Update: Celebrity, Publicity, and Branding in the Social Media Age*. New Haven, CT: Yale University Press.

Matanle, Peter, Anthony Rausch, and Shrinking Regions Research Group. 2011. *Japan's Shrinking Regions in the 21st Century*. Amherst, MA: Cambria Press.

McAfee, Andrew, and Erik Brynjolfsson. 2017. *Machine, Platform, Crowd: Harnessing Our Digital Future*. New York: W.W. Norton.

METI (Ministry of Economy, Trade, and Industry). 2010. "Special Focus: kurashi wo yutaka ni suru robotto-tachi" [Special Focus: robots for better living]." *METI Journal* 1/2 (January/February).

METI (Ministry of Economy, Trade, and Industry). 2017. "Revision of the Priority Areas to Which Robot Technology Is to Be Introduced in Nursing Care." https://www.meti.go.jp/english/press/2017/1012_002.html.

MEXT (Ministry of Education, Culture, Sports, Science and Technology). 2015. *White Paper on Science and Technology* [Tokushū ni: heisei 27-nenpan kagakugijutsu hakusho]. http://www.koho2.mext.go.jp/189/voice/189_T02.html).

Mindell, David A. 2002. *Between Human and Machine: Feedback, Control, and Computing Before Cybernetics*. Baltimore: Johns Hopkins University Press.

Miura Yoshikazu. 2014. "Panasonikku no kaigo robobeddo-kata ni mieru honkido" [The commitment behind Panasonic's robot bed for nursing care]. *Nihon keizai shimbun, denshiban*, May 19. https://www.nikkei.com/article/DGXNASDZ15 00C_V10C14A5000000/.

Miyake, Yoshiko. 1991. "Doubling Expectations: Motherhood and Women's Factory Work under State Management in Japan in the 1930s and 1940s." In *Recreating Japanese Women, 1600–1945*, edited by Gail Lee Bernstein, 267–95. Berkeley: University of California Press.

Mol, Annemarie, Ingunn Moser, and Jeannette Pols, eds. 2010. *Care in Practice: On Tinkering in Clinics, Homes and Farms*. Bielefeld: Transcript.

Morishita Takashi and Tōru Inoue. 2016. "Interactive Bio-Feedback Therapy Using Hybrid Assistive Limbs for Motor Recovery after Stroke: Current Practice and Future Perspectives." *Neurologia Medico-Chirurgica* 56(10): 605–12.

Moyle, Wendy, Marie Cooke, Elizabeth Beattie, Cindy Jones, Barbara Klein, Glenda Cook, and Chrystal Gray. 2012. "Exploring the Effect of Companion Robots on Emotional Expression in Older Adults with Dementia: A Pilot Randomized Controlled Trial." *Journal of Gerontological Nursing* 39(5): 46–53.

Murphy, Michelle. 2017. *The Economization of Life*. Durham, NC: Duke University Press.

Murphy, Samantha. 2014. "Facebook Changes Its 'Move Fast and Break Things' Motto." https://mashable.com/2014/04/30/facebooks-new-mantra-move-fast-with-stability/.

Nafus, Dawn, ed. 2017. *Quantified: Biosensing Technologies in Everyday Life.* Cambridge, MA: MIT Press.

Nagatani Keiji, Seiga Kiribayashi, Yoshito Okada, Kazuki Otake, Kazuya Yoshida, Satoshi Tadokoro, Takeshi Nishimura, Tomoaki Yoshida, Eiji Koyanagi, Mineo Fukushima, and Shinji Kawatsuma. 2013. "Emergency Response to the Nuclear Accident at the Fukushima Daiichi Nuclear Power Plants Using Mobile Rescue Robots." *Journal of Field Robotics* 30: 44–63.

Nakajima Takashi. 2016. "Robotto sūtsu HAL ni yoru Cybernic neurorehabilitation" [Cybernic neurorehabilitation using robot suit HAL]. *Shinkei Chiryōgaku (Journal of Neurological Therapeutics)* 33(3): 396–98.

Nakamura Akemi. 2004. "Robot Suit a Culmination of Sci-fi Dreams: Creator of HAL-3 Began Career Zapping Frogs." *Japan Times*, August 13.

Nakata, Hiroko. 2012. "Upgraded Quince Robots Ready for Second Foray." *Japan Times*, January 31. www.japantimes.co.jp/news/2012/01/31/news/upgraded-quince-robots-ready-for-second-foray/.

National Diet of Japan. 2012. *The Official Report of the Fukushima Nuclear Accident Independent Investigation Commission.* Executive Summary. https://www.nirs.org/wp-content/uploads/fukushima/naiic_report.pdf.

NEDO books, ed. 2009. *RT supirittsu* [Robot technology spirits]. Kawasaki: New Energy and Industrial Technology Development Organization.

Neff, Gina, and David Stark. 2004. "Permanently Beta: Responsive Organization in the Internet Era." In *Society Online: The Internet in Context,* edited by Philip E.N. Howard and Steve Jones, eds., 173–88. Thousand Oaks, CA: Sage.

Neveling, Patrick. 2018. "Export Processing Zones/Special Economic Zones." In *The International Encyclopedia of Anthropology,* edited by Hilary Callan, 2179–85. Hoboken, NJ: Wiley Blackwell.

Neven, Louis, and Christina Leeson. 2015. "Beyond Determinism: Understanding Actual Use of Social Robots by Older People." In *Aging and the Digital Life Course,* edited by David Prendergast and Chiara Garattini, 84–102. New York: Berghahn Books.

New Atlas. 2012. "Japanese First Responders to Wear Robotic Exoskeletons." October 18. https://newatlas.com/japanese-first-responders-robotic-exoskeleton/24555/.

Noble, Safiya Umoja. 2018. *Algorithms of Oppression: How Search Engines Reinforce Racism.* New York: New York University Press.

Norgren, Tiana. 2001. *Abortion before Birth Control: The Politics of Reproduction in Postwar Japan.* Princeton, NJ: Princeton University Press.

Normile, Dennis. 2021. "Endless Cleanup." *Science* 371: 983–83.

Notestein, Fred. 1945. "Population—The Long View." In *Food for the World,* edited by Theodore W. Schultz, 36–57. Chicago: University of Chicago Press.

Nozawa, Shunsuke. 2015. "Phatic Traces: Sociality in Contemporary Japan." *Anthropological Quarterly* 88(2): 373–400.

Omran, Abdel. 1971. "The Epidemiological Transition: A Theory of the Epidemiology of Population Change." *Milbank Memorial Fund Quarterly* 49(4): 509–38.

Ong, Aihwa. 2006. *Neoliberalism as Exception: Mutations in Citizenship and Sovereignty*. Durham, NC: Duke University Press.

Onishi, Norimitsu. 2011. "'Safety Myth' Left Japan Ripe for Nuclear Crisis." *New York Times*, June 24.

Owada Naotaka. 2015. "NTT to Offer Home Aid Service Featuring Talking Robot." *Nikkei Asia*, July 29. https://asia.nikkei.com/Tech-Science/Tech/NTT-to-offer-home-aid-service-featuring-talking-robot.

Penney, Matthew. 2012. "Nuclear Nationalism and Fukushima." *Asia-Pacific Journal* 10(11/2). https://apjjf.org/2012/10/11/Matthew-Penney/3712/article.html.

Pew Research Center. 2014. "Attitudes about Aging: A Global Perspective." *Global Attitudes and Trends*. January 30. https://www.pewresearch.org/global/2014/01/30/attitudes-about-aging-a-global-perspective/.

Pfadenhauer, Michaela, and Christoph Dukat. 2015. "Robot Caregiver or Robot-Supported Caregiving? The Performative Deployment of the Social Robot PARO in Dementia Care." *International Journal of Social Robotics* 7: 393–406.

Puig de la Bellacasa, Maria. 2015. "Making Time for Soil: Technoscientific Futurity and the Pace of Care." *Social Studies of Science* 45(5): 691–716.

RAT/AAT Research Group. 2002. "RAT/AAT kenkyūkai setsuritsu ni kan shi" [Regarding the establishment of the RAT/AAT Research Group]. Unpublished report. January 28.

Robertson, Jennifer. 2002. "Blood Talks: Eugenic Modernity and the Creation of New Japanese." *History and Anthropology* 13(3): 191–216.

Robertson, Jennifer. 2007. "Robo Sapiens Japanicus: Humanoid Robots and the Posthuman Family." *Critical Asian Studies* 39(3): 369–98.

Robertson, Jennifer. 2018. *Robo Sapiens Japanicus: Robots, Gender, Family, and the Japanese Nation*. Oakland: University of California Press.

Robinson, Hayley, Bruce MacDonald, Ngaire Kerse, and Elizabeth Broadbent. 2013. "The Psychosocial Effects of a Companion Robot: A Randomized Controlled Trial." *Journal of the American Medical Directors Association* 14(9): 661–67.

Roquet, Paul. 2009. "Ambient Literature and the Aesthetics of Calm: Mood Regulation in Contemporary Japanese Fiction." *Journal of Japanese Studies* 35(1): 87–111.

Rosenblat, Alex. 2018. *Uberland: How Algorithms Are Rewriting the Rules of Work*. Oakland: University of California Press.

Rostow, W. W. 1990. *The Stages of Economic Growth: A Non-Communist Manifesto*. 3rd ed. Cambridge: Cambridge University Press.

Ruckenstein, Minna, and Natasha Dow Schüll. 2017. "The Datafication of Health." *Annual Review of Anthropology* 46: 261–78.

Šabanović, Selma. 2014. "Inventing Japan's 'Robotics Culture': The Repeated Assembly of Science, Technology, and Culture in Social Robotics." *Social Studies of Science* 44(3): 342–67.

Šabanović, Selma, Casey C. Bennett, Wan-Ling Chang, Lesa Huber. 2013. "PARO Robot Affects Diverse Interaction Modalities in Group Sensory Therapy for Older Adults with Dementia." *Proceedings of the IEEE International Conference on Rehabilitation Robotics*, pp. 1–6

Šabanović, Selma, and Wan-Ling Chang. 2016. "Socializing Robots: Constructing Robotic Sociality in the Design and Use of the Assistive Robot PARO." *AI & Society* 31: 537–51.

Saito, Tomoko, Takanori Shibata, Kazuyoshi Wada, and Kazuo Tanie. 2002. "Examination of Change of Stress Reaction by Urinary Tests of Elderly before and after Introduction of Mental Commit Robot to an Elderly Institution." *Proceedings of the 7th International Symposium on Artificial Life and Robotics* 1: 316–19.

Sakai Yasuyuki. 2011. "Japan's Decline as a Robotics Superpower: Lessons from Fukushima." *Asia-Pacific Journal* 9(24/2). https://apjjf.org/2011/9/24/Sakai-Yasuyuki/3546/article.html.

Salton, Jeff. 2009. "RIBA the Friendly Robot Nurse." *New Atlas*, September 3. https://newatlas.com/riba-robot-nurse/12693/.

Samimian-Darash, Limor. 2011. "Governing through Time: Preparing for Future Threats to Health and Security." *Sociology of Health and Illness* 33(6): 930–45.

Samimian-Darash, Limor. 2013. "Governing Future Potential Biothreats: Toward an Anthropology of Uncertainty." *Current Anthropology* 54(1): 1–22.

Samuels, Richard. 2013. "Japan's Rhetoric of Crisis: Prospects for Change after 3.11." *Journal of Japanese Studies* 39(1): 97–120.

Sankai, Yoshiyuki, Kawamura Yūichirō, Okamura Junpei, Lee Su Wong. 2000. "Study on Hybrid Power Assist System HAL-1 for Walking Aid using EMG." *Proceedings of Ibaraki District Conference*. Japan Society of Mechanical Engineering, pp. 269–70.

Schodt, Frederik L. 1988. *Inside the Robot Kingdom: Japan, Mechatronics, and the Coming Robotopia*. 1st ed. New York: Kodansha International.

Scott, James C. 1998. *Seeing Like a State: How Certain Schemes to Improve the Human Condition Have Failed*. New Haven, CT: Yale University Press.

Sczesny-Kaiser, Matthias, Silke Lissek, Oliver Höffken, Volkmar Nicolas, Renate Meindl, Mirko Aach, Thomas Schildhauer, Peter Schwenkreis, and Martin Tegenthoff. 2014. "Exoskelettales Rehabilitationstraining bei Querschnittgelähmten: Fallserie zur neuronalen Plastizität" [Exoskeletal rehabilitation in chronic spinal cord injury: Case series for neuronal plasticity]. *Trauma und Berufskrankheit (Trauma and Occupational Disease)* 16: 13–15.

Seaver, Nick. 2022. *Computing Taste: Algorithms and the Makers of Music Recommendation*. Chicago: University of Chicago Press.

Seimeitai toshi: robo-shiti kōsō [Living city: The RoboCity concept]. 2011. *Fiscal*

Year 2011 Report for the Japan Society for the Promotion of Science Committee on Frontier Research and Development Project "Developing Intelligent Robots to Realize the Human–Robot Co-existence Society." Report.

Shibata, Takanori. 2012. "Therapeutic Seal Robot as Biofeedback Medical Device: Qualitative and Quantitative Evaluations of Robot Therapy in Dementia Care." *Proceedings of the IEEE* 100(8): 2527–38.

Shibata, Takanori, and Kazuyoshi Wada. 2011. "Robot Therapy: A New Approach for Mental Healthcare of the Elderly: A Mini-Review." *Gerontology* 57(4): 378–86.

Shibata, Takanori, Kazuyoshi Wada, Yōsuke Ikeda, and Selma Šabanović. 2009. "Cross-Cultural Studies on Subjective Evaluation of a Seal Robot." *Advanced Robotics* 23(4): 443–58.

Siddiqui, Faiz. 2019. "Tesla Floats Fully Self-Driving Cars as Soon as This Year: Many Are Worried about What That Will Unleash." *Washington Post*, July 17. https://www.washingtonpost.com/technology/2019/07/17/tesla-floats-fully-self -driving-cars-soon-this-year-many-are-worried-about-what-that-will-unleash/.

Smith, Noah. 2019. "Japan Begins Experiment of Opening to Immigration." *Bloomberg Opinion.* https://www.bloomberg.com/opinion/articles/2019-05-22/ japan-begins-experiment-of-opening-to-immigration

Sommerville, Ian. 2016. *Software Engineering, Global Edition.* 10th ed. Harlow: Pearson Education UK.

Sony Corporation. 1999. *Sony Launches Four-Legged Entertainment Robot: "AIBO" Creates a New Market for Robot-Based Entertainment.* https://www.sony.net/SonyInfo/News/Press_Archive/199905/99-046/.

Srnicek, Nick. 2017. *Platform Capitalism.* Cambridge: Polity.

Statista.com. 2020. "Number of Smartphones Sold to End Users Worldwide from 2007 to 2020." https://www.statista.com/statistics/263437/global-smartphone -sales-to-end-users-since-2007/

Steinberg, Marc. 2017. "A Genesis of the Platform Concept: I-mode and Platform Theory in Japan." *Asiascape: Digital Asia* 4(3): 184–208.

Steinberg, Marc. 2019. *The Platform Economy: How Japan Transformed the Consumer Internet.* Minneapolis: University of Minnesota Press.

Stern, Joanna. 2019. "First, the Smartphone Changed, Then, Over a Decade, It Changed Us." *Wall Street Journal Online*, December 17. https://www.wsj.com/ar ticles/first-the-smartphone-changed-then-over-a-decade-it-changed-us-11576618873.

Sullivan, Mark. 2003. "The New Subjective Medicine: Taking the Patient's Point of View on Health Care and Health." *Social Science & Medicine* 56(7): 1595–604.

Suzuki, Kenta, Gouji Mito, Hiroaki Kawamoto, Yasuhisa Hasegawa, and Yoshi-yuki Sankai. 2007. "Intention-Based Walking Support for Paraplegia Patients with Robot Suit HAL." *Advanced Robotics* 21(12): 1441–69.

Svendsen, Mette, Laura Navne, Iben Gjødsbøl, and Mie Dam. 2018. "A Life Worth Living: Temporality, Care, and Personhood in the Danish Welfare State." *American Ethnologist* 45(1): 20–33.

Swearingen, Jake. 2018. "We're No Longer in Smartphone Plateau: We're in the Smartphone Decline." *New York Magazine: Intelligencer.* https://nymag.com/intelligencer/2018/12/global-u-s-growth-in-smartphone-growth-starts-to-decline.html.

Taipei Times. 2003. "Japanese Ready to Launch 'Robolegs' for Commercial Use." August 22. http://www.taipeitimes.com/News/worldbiz/archives/2003/08/22/2003064776.

Thang, Leng Leng. 2011. "Aging and Social Welfare in Japan." In *The Routledge Handbook of Japanese Culture and Society*, edited by Victoria Bestor, Theodore C. Bestor, and Akiko Yamagata, 172–85. London: Routledge.

Thompson, Warren. 1929. "Population." *American Journal of Sociology* 34(6): 959–75.

Tilley, Aaron. 2017. "SoftBank Acquires Boston Dynamics from Alphabet." *Forbes*, June 8. https://www.forbes.com/sites/aarontilley/2017/06/08/softbank-acquires-boston-dynamics-from-alphabet/?sh=d957cc31d8b7.

Toyoda Kuniyoshi. 2010. "Tsukuba City Aims at 'Robot Town.'" *Japan Spotlight*, January/February, pp. 42–43.

Traphagen, John. 2006. "Power, Family, and Filial Responsibility Related to Elder Care in Rural Japan." *Care Management Journals* 7(4): 205–12.

Traphagan, John, and John Knight, eds. 2003. *Demographic Change and the Family in Japan's Aging Society*. Albany: State University of New York Press.

Tsuneoka, Chieko. 2021. "Japan's In-Home Robot Experiment Short Circuits." *Wall Street Journal*, June 29.

Tsutsui, Takako. 2014. "Implementation Process and Challenges for the Community-Based Integrated Care System in Japan." *International Journal of Integrated Care* 14: 1–9.

Turkle, Sherry. 2011. *Alone Together: Why We Expect More from Technology and Less from Each Other*. New York: Basic Books.

Twenge, Jean. 2017. *iGen: Why Today's Super-Connected Kids Are Growing Up Less Rebellious, More Tolerant, Less Happy and Completely Unprepared for Adulthood (and What This Means for the Rest of Us)*. New York: Atria Books.

United Nations. 2001. *World Population Prospects: The 2000 Revision*. New York: United Nations.

University of Tsukuba. 2017. *University of Tsukuba Admissions Guide*. http://www.human.tsukuba.ac.jp/education/wp-content/uploads/cc9536f41c0ae9662360e1f7dacfe854.pdf.

Vastag, Brian. 2011. "Robots Designed to Deal with Nuclear Accidents Await Duty in Europe While Japan Asks: Where Are Ours?" *Washington Post*, March 27. https://www.washingtonpost.com/national/robots-designed-to-deal-with-nuclear-accidents-await-duty-in-europe-while-japan-asks-where-are-ours/2011/03/25/AF2A3ClB_story.html.

Vincent, James. 2019. "Report: Boston Dynamics' Robots Are Preparing to Leave the Lab—Is the World Ready?" *The Verge*, July 7. https://www.theverge.com/2019/7/17/20697540/boston-dynamics-robots-commercial-real-world-business-spot-on-sale.

Vogt, Gabriele, and Anne-Sophie L. König. 2021. "Robotic Devices and ICT in Long-Term Care in Japan: Their Potential and Limitations from a Workplace Perspective." *Contemporary Japan*, 1–21. https://www.tandfonline.com/doi/full/10.1080/18692729.2021.2015846.

Wada, Kazuyoshi, and Kaoru Inoue, eds. 2010. *Caregiver's Manual for Robot Therapy: Practical Use of Therapeutic Seal Robot Paro in Elderly Facilities.* Tokyo: Tokyo Metropolitan University.

Wada, Kazuyoshi, and Shibata Takanori. 2007. "Living with Seal Robots: Its Sociopsychological and Physiological Influences on the Elderly at a Care House." *IEEE Transactions on Robotics* 23: 972–80.

Wada, Kazuyoshi, and Shibata Takanori. 2008. "Social and Physiological Influences of Living with Seal Robots in an Elderly Care House for Two Months." *Gerontechnology* 7(2): 235.

Wada, Kazuyoshi, Shibata Takanori, and Kawaguchi Yukitaka. 2009. "Long-Term Robot Therapy in a Health Service Facility for the Aged: A Case Study for 5 Years." *IEEE International Conference on Rehabilitation Robotics*, pp. 930–33.

Wada, Kazuyoshi, Takanori Shibata, Tomoko Saito, and Kazuo Tanie. 2002a. "Robot Assisted Activity for Elderly People and Nurses at a Day Service Center." *Proceedings of the 2002 IEEE International Conference on Robotics and Automation.* Washington, DC. May, pp. 1416–21.

Wada, Kazuyoshi, Takanori Shibata, Tomoko Saito, and Kazuo Tanie. 2002b. "Analysis of Factors that Bring Mental Effects to Elderly People in Robot-Assisted Activity." *Proceedings of the 2002 IEEE/RSJ International Conference on Intelligent Robots and Systems EPFL.* Lausanne, Switzerland, October, pp. 1152–57.

Wada, Kazuyoshi, Takanori Shibata, Toshimitsu Musha, and Shin Kimura. 2005a. "Effects of Robot Therapy for Demented Patients Evaluated by EEG." In *Proceedings of the 2005 IEEE/RSJ International Conference on Intelligent Robots and Systems*, pp. 1552–57.

Wada, Kazuyoshi, Takanori Shibata, Tomoko Saito, Kayako Sakamoto, and Kazuo Tanie. 2005b. "Psychological and Social Effects of 1-Year Robot-Assisted Activity on Elderly People at a Health Service Facility for the Aged." In *Proceedings of the 2005 IEEE International Conference on Robotics and Automation*, pp. 2785–90.

Wada, Kazuyoshi, Takanori Shibata, Tomoko Saito, Kayoko Sakamoto, and Kazuo Tanie. 2005c. "Robot-Assisted Activity at a Health Service Facility for the Aged for 17 Months: An Interim Report of Long-Term Experiment." In *Proceedings of the 2005 IEEE Workshop on Advanced Robotics and its Social Impacts*, pp. 127–32.

Wagner, Cosima. 2010. "'Silver Robots' and 'Robotic Nurses?': Japanese Robot Culture and Elderly Care." In *Demographic Change in Japan and the EU: Comparative Perspectives*, edited by Annette Schad-Seifert and Shingo Shimada, 131–54. Düsseldorf: Düsseldorf University Press.

Wedderburn, Alister. 2020. "Pandemic Time." *Soundings: A Journal of Politics and Culture* 75: 31–35.

Weng, Yueh-Hsuan, Yusuke Sugahara, Kenji Hashimoto, and Atsuo Takanishi. 2015. "Intersection of 'Tokku' Special Zone, Robots, and the Law: A Case Study on Legal Impacts to Humanoid Robots." *International Journal of Social Robotics* 7(5): 841–57.

White, Curtis. 2015. *We, Robots: Staying Human in the Age of Big Data*. Brooklyn: Melville House.

White, Merry. 2002. *Perfectly Japanese: Making Families in an Era of Upheaval*. Berkeley: University of California Press.

WHO Constitution. 1948. https://www.who.int/governance/eb/who_constitution_en.pdf.

Wiener, Norbert. 1948. *Cybernetics: Or Control and Communication in the Animal and the Machine*. Cambridge, MA: Technology Press and John Wiley.

Wiener, Norbert. 1950. *The Human Use of Human Beings: Cybernetics and Society*. Boston: Houghton Mifflin.

Wilf, Eitan. 2013. "Toward an Anthropology of Computer-Mediated, Algorithmic Forms of Sociality." *Current Anthropology* 54(6): 716–39.

Wilf, Eitan. 2019. "Separating Noise from Signal: The Ethnomethodological Uncanny as Aesthetic Pleasure in Human–Machine Interaction in the United States." *American Ethnologist* 46: 202–13.

Winance, Myriam. 2010. "Care and Disability: Practices of Experimenting, Tinkering With, and Arranging People and Technical Aids." In *Care in Practice: On Tinkering in Clinics, Homes and Farms*, edited by Annemarie Mol, Ingunn Moser, and Jeannette Pols, 93–117. Bielefeld: Transcript.

Winner, Langdon. 1980. "Do Artifacts Have Politics?" *Daedalus* 109(1): 121–36.

Wolkomir, Richard. 1985. "The Machine Servant." In *Robotics*, edited by Marvin Minsky, 214–35. New York: Anchor Press/Doubleday.

World Bank. 1994. *Averting the Old Age Crisis: Policies to Protect the Old and Promote Growth*. Oxford University Press: Oxford. http://www-wds.worldbank.org/ servlet/WDSContentServer/WDSP/IB/199 4/09/01/000009265_3970311 123336/ Rendered/PDF/multi_page.pdf.

World Bank. 2023. "Population Ages 65 and Above (% of Total Population)— Germany." *World Bank Group*. https://data.worldbank.org/indicator/SP.POP.65UP.TO.ZS?locations=DE.

World Bank. 2024. "Population Ages 65 and Above (% of Total Population)— Japan." *World Bank Group*. https://data.worldbank.org/indicator/SP.POP.65UP.TO.ZS?locations=JP.

Wright, James. 2021. "Overcoming Political Distrust: The Role of 'Self-Restraint' in Japan's Public Health Response to COVID-19." *Japan Forum* 33(4): 453–75.

Wright, James. 2023. *Robots Won't Save Japan: An Ethnography of Eldercare Automation*. Ithaca, NY: Cornell University Press.

Yamada, Minoru, and Hidenori Arai. 2020. "Long-Term Care System in Japan." *Annals of Geriatric Medicine and Research* 24(3): 174–80.

Yashiro, Naohiro. 2005. "Japan's New Special Zones for Regulatory Reform." *International Tax and Public Finance* 12: 561–74.

Yokoyama Kazuhiko. 2004. "Robotto shitī ni mukete no RT yunitto to RT konpōnento" [RT units and RT components in Robot City]. *Nihon robotto gakkai-shi* 22(7): 843–46.

Young, Louise. 1998. *Japan's Total Empire: Manchuria and the Culture of Wartime Imperialism*. Berkeley: University of California Press.

Zaloom, Caitlin. 2004. "The Productive Life of Risk." *Cultural Anthropology* 19(3): 365–91.

Zhan, Mei. 2009. *Other-Worldly: Making Chinese Medicine through Transnational Frames*. Durham, NC: Duke University Press.

Zuboff, Shoshana. 2020. *The Age of Surveillance Capitalism: The Fight for a Human Future at the New Frontier of Power*. New York: Public Affairs.

INDEX

Page numbers in italics denote figures. Endnotes are indicated by "n" followed by the endnote number.

The authorized representative in the EU for product safety and compliance is:
Mare Nostrum Group
B.V Doelen 72
4831 GR Breda
The Netherlands

www.ingramcontent.com/pod-product-compliance
Lightning Source LLC
Chambersburg PA
CBHW030401270326
41926CB00009B/1208